Pharmaceutical Word Book

Barbara De Lorenzo
Medical Transcriptionist
Toms River, New Jersey

1985
W. B. Saunders Company
Philadelphia London Toronto Mexico City
Rio de Janeiro Sydney Tokyo

W. B. Saunders Company: West Washington Square
                           Philadelphia, PA 19105

                           1 St. Anne's Road
                           Eastbourne, East Sussex BN21 3UN, England

                           1 Goldthorne Avenue
                           Toronto, Ontario M8Z 5T9, Canada

                           Apartado 26370—Cedro 512
                           Mexico 4, D.F., Mexico

                           Rua Coronel Cabrita, 8
                           Sao Cristovao Caixa Postal 21176
                           Rio de Janeiro, Brazil

                           9 Waltham Street
                           Artarmon, N.S.W. 2064, Australia

                           Ichibancho, Central Bldg., 22-1 Ichibancho
                           Chiyoda-Ku, Tokyo 102, Japan

Library of Congress Cataloging in Publication Data

De Lorenzo, Barbara.
Pharmaceutical word book.

1. Drugs—Dictionaries.   I. Title.
RS51.D4   1985   615.1'03'21   84–22158

ISBN 0–7216–1459–0

Pharmaceutical Word Book   ISBN 0–7216–1459–0

Last digit is the print number: 9   8   7   6   5   4   3   2   1

To Mom
Who made it all possible

PREFACE

The large reference books published today are invaluable because they make available essential information on major pharmaceutical and diagnostic products.

There are many instances, however, when the spelling and not the meaning of a word is in doubt. Considerable time could be saved if the professional were able to consult only one compact text rather than a large number of heavy volumes containing drug listings. I searched for a text prepared for those who needed a simple, accurate, up-to-date book containing only the spelling of generic and trade drug names, and clearly indicating capitalization where necessary. The tests I came across were large, bulky reference books.

This text is designed to provide an easy to use, handy, thorough, word book that serves the needs of a varied audience in the health sciences. It contains thousands of drug entries, both generic and trade names, and it is alphabetically arranged with capitalization or lower case clearly shown. American spellings are used throughout, but British spellings are also included and are marked by a raised dot preceding the entry. This text is inexpensive and compact and will be an invaluable desk reference for anyone involved in transcribing, editing, teaching, or recording material that includes medical terminology. The format of merely listing spelling and clearly marking capitalization, where required, provides a time-saving aid and a quick reference guide for persons interested in verifying only spelling.

B. DE LORENZO

ACKNOWLEDGMENTS

I am deeply grateful to all those who have given me the opportunity to learn, particularly Doris Fedun, R.N., who inspired me.

I would like to express my sincere appreciation to the staff of W. B. Saunders, especially Baxter Venable and his assistant Debra Vickery. I would also like to acknowledge Joe Dixon for his expert guidance in the computer field.

I am most especially grateful to my family and friends for their support and encouragement.

A

A-200 Pyrinate
A-A Comp Tablets
AAS
Abbocillin
Abbokinase
ABCDG Vitamin Capsules
Abdec Baby Vitamin Drops
Abdec Kapseals
Abdol
Abminthic
Absorbine
Abuscreen
A.C.A. No. 4
A.C.A. No. 5
A-Caine
A-Caps
Acarbose
Accelerase
Accelerase-PB
Accurbron
Accutane
A.C.D. Capsules
Ac-Di-Sol
A-C-D Solution
acebutolol
acecainide hydrochloride
aceclidine
acedapsone

Acedoval
Acedyne
•acefluranol
Acelax
•acemetacin
A'Cenol
Acephen
•acepifylline
acepromazine maleate
Acerola-C
Acerola-Plex
Aceta
Acetabar
Aceta-Gesic
acetamide
acetaminophen
•acetarsol
acetarsone
Acetasem
acetazolamide sodium
Acetest
acetic acid
acetohexamide
acetohydroxamic acid
Acetojen Jr.
Acetolax
acetomeroctol
acetone

1

acetophenazine maleate
•acetorphine
Acetospan
acetosulfone sodium
Acetotot
acetrizoate sodium
acetrizoic acid
acetylcarbromal
acetylcholine chloride
acetylcysteine (n-
  acetylcysteine)
acetyldigitoxin
acetyltannic acid
Achromycin
Achromycin V
Achrostatin V
Acid Mantle
Acidol-Pepsin
Acidoride
Acidulin
Aci-Jel
Acillin
•acinitrazole
Aciquel
acivicin
aclarubicin
•aclatonium napadisilate
Acnaveen
Acne-Aid
Acnederm
Acne-Dome
Acnesarb
Acno
Acnomel
Acnophill
Acnotex
A.C.N. Tablets
acodazole hydrochloride

Acon
Acotus
ACR
acrisorcin
acronine
•acrosoxacin
ACT
Actacin
Actagen
Actamin
actaplanin
Actase
ACTH: adrenocorticotropin
Acthar
Acticort
Actidil
Acti-Dione
Actif VIII
Actifed
Actifed-C
Actihist
actinomycotin
actinoquinol sodium
Acti-Prem
actodigin
Actol
Actrapid
Actylate
ACU-dyne
Acupan
Acutran
Acutrim
acyclovir
Acylanid
Adalin
Adanon
Adapettes
Adapin

Adapt
Adatuss
Adavite
Adavite-M
Adeflor
Adeflor M
Ademol
Adeno
adenosine phosphate
Adequate Improved Tablets
•adicillin
Adipex-P
adiphenine hydrochloride
Adphen
A-D-R
Adrenalin
adrenalone
Adrenatrate
adrenocorticotropic
   hormone: ACTH
Adrenoscan
Adrestat F
Adriamycin
Adroyd
Adrucil
Adsorbocarpine
Adsorbonac
Adsorbotear
Adsormone
Advance
Advent
Aerdil
aeroCAINE
Aerodine
Aerohalor
Aerolate
Aeroseb-Dex
Aeroseb-HC

Aerosept
Aerosporin
Aerosporin Otic
aeroTHERM
Afaxin
A-Fil
Afko-Lube
Afrikol
Afrin
Afrinol
Aftate
Agoral
A/G-Pro
Agribon
Ahan
A-hydroCort
Aidant
Aid-Tuss
Airet GG II
Airet LA
Air-Tabs G.G.
Akarpine
Ak-Cide
Ak-Con
Ak-Dex
Ak-Dilate
Akes-N-Pain
Ak-Fluor
Akineton
aklomide
Akne Drying Lotion
Ak-Nefrin
Ak-Neo-Cort
Akoline
Akoline C.B.
Ak-Pentolate
Ak-Pred
Akrinol

Ak-Rinse
Ak-Sulf
Ak-Sulf Forte
Ak-Taine
Ak-Tate
Akwa Tears
Ak-Zol
Ala-Cort
Aladrine
Alamag
alamecin
Alamine
Alamine-C
alanine
alaproclate
Ala-Quin
Ala-Tet
Alaxin
AL-AY
Alazide
Albalon
Alba-Natal
Albay
albendazole
albumin, aggregated
albumin, aggregated
   iodinated I-131 serum
albumin, chromated Cr 51
   serum
albumin human
albumin, iodinated I-125
Albuminar
Albumisol
Albumotope I-125
Albumotope I-131
Albumotope-LS
Albuspan
Albutein

albuterol
   a. sulfate
albutoin
Alcaine
Alcare
alclofenac
alclometasone dipropionate
alcloxa
alcohol
   absolute a.
   amyl a.
   amyl a., tertiary
   anisyl a.
   aromatic a.
   azeotropic isopropyl a.
   batyl a.
   benzyl a.
   bornyl a.
   butyl a.
   camphyl a.
   carnaubyl a.
   ceryl a.
   cetyl a.
   cinnamyl a.
   dehydrated a.
   denatured a.
   deodorized a.
   dihydric a.
   diluted a.
   ethyl a.
   fatty a.
   glyceryl a., glycyl a.
   isoamyl a.
   isobutyl a.
   isopropyl a.
   isopropyl rubbing a.
   ketone a.
   lanolin a's.

Alcohol *(continued)*
   methyl a.
   monohydric a.
   nicotinyl a.
   palmityl a.
   pantothenyl a.
   phenylethyl a.
   phenylic a.
   polyglucosic a.
   polyvinyl a.
   primary a.
   n-propyl a.
   rubbing a.
   secondary a.
   stearyl a.
   sugar a's.
   tertiary a.
   tribromoethyl a.
   trihydric a.
   unsaturated a.
   wood a.
Alcojet
Alcolec
Alconefrin
Alconox
Alco-Vite
alcuronium chloride
Aldactazide
Aldactone
aldioxa
Aldoclor
Aldomet
Aldoril
•aldosterone
Alermine
Alersule
aletamine hydrochloride
Aleuronat

alexidine
•alexitol sodium
alfaprostol
Alfavet
Alfenta
algeldrate
Algemol
Algenic Alka
algestone acetonide
algestone acetophenide
Algetuss
Algin-All
aliflurane
•alinidine
alipamide
Alka-Med
Alka-Seltzer
Alkeran
Alkets
allantoin
Allbee C-800
Allbee w/C
Allbee-T
Aller-Chlor
Allercreme
Allerest
Allerform
Allerfrin
Allergan Hydrocare
Allergesic
Allergine
Allerid-D.C.
Allerid-O.D.
Allerprop
Allersone
Allerspan
Allerstat
•alletorphine

allobarbital
Alloferin
allopurinol
Allpyral
•allyloestrenol
•allyprodine
Almacone
almadrate sulfate
Alma-Mag
Alma-Mag #4
Almocarpine
Almora
Alnovin
Alnyte
aloe
alofilcon A
alonimid
Alophen
Alorain
Alo-Tuss
•aloxidone
•aloxiprin
alpertine
alpha amylase
•alphacetylmethadol
Alpha Chymar
alpha chymotrypsin
Alphacne
Alphaderm
•alphadolone
Alphadrol
Alpha Keri
Alphalin
•alphameprodine
Alphamin
Alphamul
alphanaphthol
alphaprodine hydrochloride

alphaREDISOL
Alpha-Ruvite
•alphaxalone
Alphosyl
Alphosyl-HC
alprazolam
alprenolol hydrochloride
alprostadil
alrestatin sodium
alseroxylon
Altafur
Altapin
ALternaGEL
Altex
Altexide
althiazide
altrenogest
Alucaine
Alu-Cap
Al-U-Creme
Aludrox
alum
Alumadrine
Alumid
aluminum acetate
    a. chloride hexahydrate
    a. chlorohydrate
    a. chlorohydrex
    a. glycinate
    a. hydroxide
    a. phosphate
    a. sesquichlorohydrate
    a. subacetate
    a. sulfate
    a. zirconium tetra-
        chlorohydrex Gly
    a. zirconium trichloro-
        hydrex Gly

Alupent
Alurate
Alurex
Aluscop
Alu-Tab
AluWets
Alvagel
Alvedil
Alveograf
alverine citrate
Al-Vite
amadinone acetate
amantadine hydrochloride
Amaphen
Amaril D
Amaril D Spantabs
Ambay
•ambazone
ambenonium chloride
•ambenoxan
Ambenyl
Amberlite
•ambicromil
Ambodryl
ambomycin
Ambrine
ambruticin
ambuphylline
ambuside
ambutoxate hydrochloride
AMC
Amcap
Am-Ch
Amcill
amcinafal
amcinafide
amcinonide
Amcort

amdinocillin
    a. pivoxil
amedalin hydrochloride
Amen
Americaine
Amertan
Amesec
ametantrone acetate
•ametazole hydrochloride
A-MethaPred
amethocaine hydrochloride
amfenac sodium
amfonelic acid
Amforol
Amicar
•amicarbalide
amicloral
amicycline
amidapsone
Amidate
amidephrine mesylate
Amide-VC
Amide V/S
Amidoxine
Amid-Sal
Amifur
Amigen
Amijex 1250
amikacin sulfate
Amikin
amiloride hydrochloride
aminacrine hydrochloride
Amin-Aid
Aminess
aminitrozole
aminoacetic acid
Aminobrain PT
aminocaproic acid

Aminodur
aminoglutethimide
aminohippurate sodium
aminohippuric acid
•aminometradine
aminopentamide sulfate
aminophylline
Aminoprel
•aminopterin sodium
aminopyrine
aminorex
aminosalicylate calcium
   a. potassium
   a. sodium
aminosalicylic acid
Aminosol
Aminosyn
Aminosyn R.F.
aminotrate
   a. phosphate
Amipaque
amiquinsin hydrochloride
Amiron
Amitid
Amitin
Amitone
amitraz
Amitril
amitriptyline hydrochloride
ammonia, aromatic spirit
ammoniated mercury
ammonium benzoate
   a. carbonate
   a. chloride
   a. mandelate
   a. phosphate
   a. tartrate
   a. valerate

Amnioplastin
Amniotin
amobarbital sodium
Amobell
Amocal Jr.
Amocillin
Amocine
Amo-Derm
Amodex
amodiaquine hydrochloride
Amodin
Amodrine
Amoebicon
Amogel
Amoline
Amonidrin
amopyroquin hydrochloride
Amosan
amoxapine
amoxicillin
Amoxil
Amphaplex
amphecloral
Amphenol
amphetamine sulfate
Amphojel
amphomycin
amphotericin B
ampicillin
•amprolium
amprotropine phosphate
ampyzine sulfate
amquinate
amrinone
amsacrine
Amstat
Amsustain
A-M-T

Amvisc
amylene hydrate
amyl nitrite
•amylmetacresol
•amylobarbitone
Amytal
Anabol
Anabolin LA-100
Anabolin I.M.
Anacel
Anacin
Anacin-3
Anadrol
Anadrol-50
Anafed
anagestone acetate
anagrelide hydrochloride
Analbalm
Analgesine
Analone-50
Anamine
Ananase
Anaphen
Anaprox
Anaspaz
Anaspaz PB
Anavar
anazolene sodium
Anbesol
Ancef
Ancobon
ancrod
Andoin
Andrenex
Andrest 90-4
Andriol
Andro 100
Andro L.A.

Andro L.A.200
Andro-Cyp 100
Andro/Fem
Androgyn L.A.
Android
Android-F
Android-HCG
Android-T
Android-10
Androlone
Androlone-D 50
Andronate 100
Andryl
Anduracaine
Anectine
Anectine Flo-Pak
Anergan 25
Anestacon
Anesthesin
anethole
Anexsia
Angex
Angio-Conray
angiotensin amide
Angiovist
Angitab
Angitrate
Ang-O-Span
Anhydron
anidoxime
A-Nil
anileridine
anilopam hydrochloride
aniracetam
anise oil
anisindione
anisotropine methylbromide
anitrazafen

Anocaine
Anodynos
Anoquan
Anorex
Anorexin
anoxomer
Ansaid
Ansemco No. 2
Anspor
Antabuse
antazoline phosphate
Antepar
Anthatest
anthelmycin
Anthra-Derm
anthralin
anthramycin
anthraquinone
Anti-B
Antibiopto
Anti-Chlor
Antifebrin
Antilirium
Antiminth
antimony potassium tartrate
   a. trisulfide colloid
Anti-N Lectin
antipyrine
Antispas
Anti-Ten
Anti-Therm
Antitrem
Anti-Tuss
antivenin (crotalidae)
  polyvalent
Antivert
Antrenyl
Antrocol

Antuitrin S
Anturane
Anucaine
Anugard-HC
Anuject
Anuphen
Anusol
Anusol-HC
Anyage
APAC
Apatate
apazone
A.P.B.
A.P.C.
Apcogesic
Apcohist
Apcoretic
Aphonal
A.P.L.
Aplisol
Aplitest
Apogen
apomorphine
A-Poxide
Appedrine
Appet-Aid
Appet-Iron
Appress
apramycin
Apresazide
Apresodex
Apresoline
aprindine hydrochloride
aprobarbital
aprotinin
Aptine
•aptocaine
Aqua-Ban

Aquabase
Aquacare
Aquacycline
Aquaderm
Aqua-Film Tears
Aquaflex
Aqua Ivy
AquaMEPHYTON
Aquamycin
Aquaphilic
Aquaphor
Aquaphyllin
Aqua-Scrip
Aquasec
Aquasol A
Aquasol E
Aquatag
Aquatensen
Aquest
Aquex
Aralen
Aramine
aranotin
arbaprostil
Arbon
Arcobee
Arco-Cee
Arco-Lase
Arco-Lase Plus
Arcoret
Arco-Thyroid
Arcotinic
Arcum R-S
Arcum V-M
Arcylate
A-R-D
Ardeben
Ardecaine

Ardefem
Arfonad
Argesic
arginine glutamate
    a. hydrochloride
argipressin tannate
Argyrol
Argyrol S.S.
arildone
Aristocort
Aristocort Acetonide
Aristocort Forte
Aristospan
Arlacel C
Arlamol E
Arlidin
A.R.M. Tablets
Arpocox
arprinocid
Arquel
arsanilic acid
arsphenamine
Artane
artegraft
Arthralgen
Arthrolate
Arthropan
Articulose L.A.
Articulose 50
A.S.A.
Asalco No. 1, No. 2
A.S.B.
Asbron G
ascorbic acid
Ascorbicap
Ascriptin
Asellacrin
Asendin

Asmalix
Asmatane Mist
Asminyl
Asminorel
Asmolin
asparaginase
asparagine
aspartame
aspartic acid
aspartocin
Asperbuf
Aspercreme
Aspergum
asperlin
Asphac-G
Aspirbar
aspirin
Aspirjen Jr.
Aspir-Phen
Aspirtab
Aspodyne
Asproject
astemizole
Asthmacon
AsthmaHaler
AsthmaNefrin
Astring-O-Sol
astromicin sulfate
Astro-Vites
Atabee TD
Atabrine
Atarax
Ataraxoid
atenolol
Atgam
Atgard
Atgard C
Atgard V

Athemol
Athrombin-K
Ativan
atolide
Atpeg 400
atracurium besylate
Atridine
Atrobarb No. 1, No. 2,
    No. 3
Atrocap
Atrocholin
Atromid-S
atropine
    a. oxide hydrochloride
    a. sulfate
Atropisol
Atrosed
Atrovent
A/T/S
Attenuvax
Auralgan
auranofin
Aureomycin
Auristil
Auri-Tuss
Aurocaine
Auro-Dri
Auro Ear Drops
Auromid
aurothioglucose
Ausab
Aus-Tect
Austigen
Autoplex
A-Van
Avatec
Avazyme
AVC

Aveeno
Aventyl
Aventyl HCl
Avertin
Avicel
A-Vitan
Avitene
Avlosulfon
avoparcin
Axotal
Axsinate
Ayds AM/PM
Aygestin
Ayr
azabon
azacitidine
azaclorzine hydrochloride
azaconazole
azacosterol hydrochloride
•azalomycin
•azamethonium bromide
azanator maleate
azanidazole
azaperone
•azapropazone
azaribine
azarole
azaserine

azatadine maleate
azathioprine
Azene
azepindole
azetepa
•azidocillin
azipramine hydrochloride
Azlin
azlocillin
Azma Aid
Azmacort
Azodine
Azo Gantanol
Azo Gantrisin
Azolid
Azolid-A
azolimine
Azo-Pyridon
azosemide
Azo-Soxazole
Azo-Standard
Azo-Stat
Azo-Sulfisoxazole
Azo-Sulfizin
azotomycin
Azotrex
aztreonam
Azulfidine

B

B-A
bacampicillin hydrochloride
Bacarate
Bacid
Baciguent

Bacimycin
bacitracin
baclofen
Bactal Soap
Bactalin

Bact-Chek
Bactine
Bactocill
Bactrim
Bactrim DS
Bafil
BAL in Oil
•balipramine
Balmex
Balneol
Balnetar
•balsalazide
balsam of Peru
Baltron
Bamadex
Bamate
bamethan sulfate
bamifylline hydrochloride
•bamipine
bamnidazole
Banalg
Banatil
Bancaps
bandage, adhesive
bandage, gauze
Ban-Drowz
Banesin
Banflex
Banminth
Banthine
Barachlor
Barazole
Barbeloid
Barbidonna
Barbinal
Barbipil
Barbita
barbital

•barbitone
Barc gel, liquid, spray
Bar-Cy-Amine
Bar-Cy-A-Tab
Baridium
Bari-Stress
Baritrate
barium hydroxide lime
    b. sulfate
Barlevite
Barodense
Baroflave
Barogel
Baroloid
Barophen
Barosperse
Barotrast
Barotussin
Barovite
Barseb HC
Barseb Thera-Spray
Bar-Test
Bartone
Bar-Tropin
Basa
Basaljel
Baselan
Baumodyne Gel
Baximin
Baxinets
Bayaminic
Bayaminicol
Bayapap
Bay-Ase
Baycodan
Baycomine
Baycotussend
Baydec DM

Bayer
Bayfrin
Bayhistine
Baylox
Baymethazine
Bayon
Bay-Ornade
Baytussin
Baytussin DM
B-C-Bid Capsules
B-C-E
BC Tablets
BC-Vite
becanthone hydrochloride
Because
Be-Ce-Forte
Be-Ce-Plex
•beclamide
•beclobrate
beclomethasone dipropionate
Beclovent
Becomco
Becomject-100
Beconase
Becoplex
Becotin-T
Becotin w/C
Becozym
Bedoce
Bedoce-Gel
Bee-Forte
Beelith
Beepen-VK
Beesix
Bee-T-Vites
Bee-Zee Tabs
Bejectal
Belap

Belexal
Belfer
Bellachar
Belladenal
Belladenal-S
belladonna
    b. alkaloids
Bellafoline
Bellalphen
Bellaneed
Bell/ans
Bellergal
Bellergal-S
Bellkatal
Bellophen
beloxamide
bemegride
•bemetizide
Bemex
Beminal-500
Beminal Forte
Bena-D
Benadryl
Benadyne
Benahist
benapryzine hydrochloride
Benase
Benasept
Ben-Aqua-5
bendazac
Bendectin
Bendopa
bendroflumethiazide
Bendylate
•benethamine penicillin
Benegyn
Benemid
Ben-Gay

Benisone
Benoject
Benoquin
Benoral
benorterone
benorylate
benoxaprofen
benoxinate hydrochloride
Benoxyl
benperidol
bensalan
benserazide
•bensuldazic acid
Bensulfoid
bentazepam
Bentical
bentiromide
bentonite
Bentyl
benurestat
Benylate
Benylin
Benylin DM
Benzac
Benzac W
Benzagel
benzaldehyde
benzalkonium chloride
benzathine penicillin G
benzazoline hydrochloride
benzbromarone
Benz-Ease
Benzedrex
Benzedrine
benzestrol
benzethonium chloride
benzetimide hydrochloride
•benzhexol

benzilonium bromide
benzindopyrine
   hydrochloride
•benziodarone
Benzo-C
benzocaine
Benzocol
benzoctamine hydrochloride
Benzodent
benzodepa
benzodiazepine
Benzodyne
benzoic acid
benzoin
benzonatate
Benzopropyl
benzoxiquine
benzoyl peroxide
benzoylpas calcium
benzphetamine
benzquinamide
benzthiazide
benztropine mesylate
benzydamine hydrochloride
benzyl alcohol
benzyl benzoate
benzylpenicillin
bephenium
   hydroxynaphthoate
bepridil hydrochloride
Ber-Ex
Bergotal
Berocca
Berocca-C
Berocca-PN
Berocca-WS
Bersotrin
Berubigen

berythromycin
Besan
Besaprin
Beserol
Besitex B1
Besta
Best-C
Bestrone
Beta-B-Plex
beta carotene
Betacrest
Betaderm
Betadine
betahistine hydrochloride
Betalin S
Betalin 12 Crystalline
Betalin Complex
Betalin Compound
Betalin S
Beta-2
•betameprodine
•betamethadol
betamethasone
    b. acetate
    b. benzoate
    b. dipropionate
    b. sodium phosphate
    b. valerate
betamicin sulfate
Betapen-VK
•betaprodine
Betaprone
Betatrex
Beta-Val
Beta-Vite
Betaxin
betaxolol hydrochloride
betazole hydrochloride

bethanechol chloride
bethanidine sulfate
Betuline
bevantolol hydrochloride
Bevatine-12
Bevidox
Bewon
Bexibee
Bexo-C
Bexomal-C
bezafibrate
bezalip
•bezitramide
B.F.I. Antiseptic
bialamicol hydrochloride
Biamine
Biarsan
Biavax-II
•bibenzonium bromide
bicifadine hydrochloride
Bicillin
Bicillin C-R
Bicillin L-A
Bicitra
•bidimazium iodide
•bifluranol
bifonazole
Bi-K
Bilagog
Bilamide
Bilax
Bilechol
Bilezyme
Bilezyme Plus
Bilitec
Bilogen
Bilopaque
Biloric

Bilron
Biltricide
Binex-C
biniramycin
Bio-Crest
Bio-des
Bio/Dopa
Bioepiderm
bioflavonoids
Biopar Forte
Bioslim T
Biosone
Bio-Sorb
biotin
Biotres
Biozyme-C
biperiden hydrochloride
    b. lactate
biphenamine hydrochloride
Biphetamine
Bipole-S
Bironate-B
bisacodyl
    b. tannex
Bisalate
bisantrene hydrochloride
Biscolan
Bisco-Lax
bismuth aluminate
    b. betanaphthol
    b. citrate
    b. cream
    •b. glycollylarsanilate
    b. magma
    b. potassium tartrate
    b. sodium
      triglycollamate
    b. subcarbonate

bismuth (*continued*)
    b. subgallate
    b. subnitrate
    b. subsalicylate
bisobrin lactate
•bisoprolol
Bisodol
bisoxatin acetate
Bisquadine
bithionolate sodium
bitolterol mesylate
Bitrex
Black-Draught
Blaintrate
Blanex
Blaud Strubel
blastomycin
Blenoxane
bleomycin sulfate
Blephamide
Bleph-10 Liquifilm
Bleph-10 S.O.P.
Blephamide S.O.P.
Blink-N-Clean
Blinx
Blis
Blistaid
Blistex
Blis-To-Sol
Bloat Guard
Blocadren
Block-Aid
Blockain HCl
Block Out
Bluboro
Bludex
Blu-Hist
Blupav

B-Major
B.M.E.
B-N
B-Nutron
B and O Supprettes
Bo-Car-Al
Boil-Ease
Boil n Soak
bolandiol dipropionate
bolasterone
Bolax
boldenone undecylenate
bolenol
bolmantalate
Bon-A-Day
Bonaid
Bonine
Bonomycin
Bon-O-Tin
Bontril PDM
Bopen-VK
boric acid
•bornaprine
bornelone
Borofax
Borosorb
botulism antitoxin
Bovatec
Bowman Cold Tablets
Bowtussin D.M.
boxidine
Boyol
BP-5
B-Pap
B-Pas
BPN
BP-Papaverine
B.P.P.-Lemmon

BPS
B.Q.R.
Brace
Brasivol
Breacol
Breatheasy
Breezee Mist
Breokinase
Breonesin
Breonex-L
Brethine
bretylium tosylate
Bretylol
Brevicon
Brevital
brewer's yeast
Brexin
Bricanyl
Brigen-G
brinolase
Bristacycline
Bristagen
Bristamycin
Bristoject
British anti-lewisite:
    BAL
Brobella-P.B.
Brocillin
Brocon C.R.
brocresine
brofezil
brofoxine
Brogesic
Brohembione
Brolade
bromadoline maleate
Bromalate
Bromalix

Bromanyl
Bromapapp
bromazepam
Bromenzyme
Bromfed
Bromfed-PD
bromhexine hydro-
   chloride
bromide
bromindione
bromocriptine mesylate
bromodiphenhydramine
   hydrochloride
Bromophen T.D.
Bromo-Seltzer
Bromotuss
bromoxanide
bromperidol
   b. decanoate
Bromphen
brompheniramine
   maleate
Bromsulphalein
Bromtapp
Bromural
Broncajen
Bronchobid Duracap
Bronchohist
Broncholate
Bronchovent
Broncol
Brondecon Tablets
Bronitin
Bronkaid
Bronkephrine
Bronkodyl
Bronkodyl S-R
Bronkolixir Elixir

Bronkometer
Bronkosol
Bronkotabs
Bronsecur
Bron-Sed
broperamole
Brophed
Broserpine
Brotane
Bro-Tapp
brotizolam
Brucellergen
Bryrel
B-Scorbic
BSS Plus
bucainide maleate
bucindolol hydro-
   chloride
Bucladin-S
buclizine hydrochloride
bucrylate
budesonide
•bufexamac
Buff-A
Buffacetin
Buff-A Comp
Buff-A Comp No.3
Buffadyne-Lemmon
Buffaprin
Bufferin
Buffets
Buffex
Buffinol
bufilcon A
BufOpto
buformin
Buf-Oxal 5
•bufrolin

Bufs
Buf-Sul
Buf-Tabs
•bufuralol
Bu-Lax 100
Bu-Lax 250
bumetanide
bumetrizole
Bumex
Buminate
bunamidine hydro-
   chloride
bunolol hydrochloride
bupicomide
bupivacaine hydrochloride
Buprenex
buprenorphine hydro-
   chloride
bupropion hydrochloride
buquinolate
buramate
Burdeo
Burn-A-Lay
Burnate
Burn-Quel
Burntame
Bur-Oil-Zinc
Buro-Sol
Burotor
Burow's Solution
Bursul
Bur-Tuss
Bur-Zin
buserelin acetate
Busone
Buspar
buspirone hydrochloride
busulfan

Butabar
butabarbital sodium
butacaine sulfate
butacetin
butaclamol hydrochloride
Butal
Butalan
butalbital
Butalix
butallylonal
butamben
   b. picrate
butamirate citrate
butamisole hydrochloride
butaperazine
   b. maleate
Butaphyllamine
Butatran
Butatrax
Butazem
Butazolidin
buterizine
Butesin
butethal
butethamine hydrochloride
buthiazide
Butibel
Butibel-Zyme
Buticaps
butikacin
butilfenin
butirosin sulfate
Butisol Sodium
butixirate
butoconazole nitrate
butonate
butopamine
butoprozine hydrochloride

butopyronoxyl
butorphanol
    b. tartrate
butoxamine hydrochloride

butriptyline hydrochloride
butylparaben
Butyn
B-Vite

C

Cabadon-M
Cabcurve Lens
cabufocon A
cabufocon B
cactinomycin
•cadexomer-iodine
Cad-O-Bath
Cadophill
Cafacetin
Cafecon
•cafedrine
Cafergot
Cafertabs
Cafetrate
caffeine
Caffin-T.D.
Cagol
Caladryl
Calaformula
Calamatum
calamine
Calamycin
Calamox
Calan
Calbrodex
Cal-C-Bate
Calcee
Calcet Tabs
Calcibind

Calcicaps Four
Calcidrine
calcifediol
Calcilac
Calcimar
Calciparine
calcitonin
calcitriol
calcium
    c. ascorbate
    c. carbonate
    c. caseinate
    c. chloride
    c. disodium edathamil
    c. disodium edetate
    c. disodium versenate
    c. edetate sodium
    c. glubionate
    c. gluconate
    c. hydroxide
    c. lactate
    c. levulinate
    c. mandelate
    c. pantothenate
    c. pantothenate,
        racemic
    c. phosphate, dibasic
    c. polycarbophil
Calciwafers

CaldeCORT
Calderol
Caldesene
Cal-D-Mint
Cal-D-Phos
Calfer-Vite
Calglycine
Calicarb
Calinate-FA
Calivite
Calmol 4
Calmosin
Calm X
Cal-Nor
calomel
Calpholac
Calphosan
Calphosan-B-12
Cal-Prenal
Calsa
Calsan
Calsarbain
Calscorbate
Cal-Sup
Caltrate 600
Caltro
calusterone
Cal-Zo
Cama Inlay-Tabs
Camalox
Cam-ap-es
cambendazole
Campho-Phenique
camphor
Candex
candicidin
Cankaid
•cannabinol

Canopar
canrenoate potassium
canrenone
cantharidin
Cantharone
Cantil
Cantri
Canz
C-A-P
Capahist
Capahist-DMH
Capastat
Capital
Capitrol
Ca-Plus
Capnitro
capobenate sodium
capobenic acid
Capoten
capreomycin sulfate
Capron
Capsebon
captamine hydrochloride
•captodiame
captopril
Capulets
capuride
Caquin
caracemide
Carafate
Carbacel
carbachol
carbadox
carbamazepine
carbamide peroxide
carbantel lauryl sulfate
carbarsone
carbaspirin calcium

carbazeran
carbazochrome salicylate
carbenicillin disodium
   c. indanyl sodium
   c. phenyl sodium
   c. potassium
carbenoxolone sodium
carbetapentane citrate
carbethyl salicylate
carbidopa
•carbimazole
carbinoxamine maleate
carbiphene hydrochloride
Carbocaine
•carbocisteine
carbocloral
carbocysteine
Carbodec DM
carbolic acid
•carbolonium bromide
carbomer 910
   c. 934
   c. 934P
   c. 940
   c. 941
carbon dioxide
carbon tetrachloride
carboplatin
Carbopol 910
   C. 934
   C. 934P
   C. 940
   C. 941
carboprost
   c. methyl
   c. tromethamine
Carb-O-Sep
Carbowax

carboxymethylcellulose
  calcium
   c. sodium
Carbrital
carbromal
carbuterol hydro-
  chloride
Cardenz
Cardiazol
Cardilate
Cardiografin
Cardio-Green
Cardioquin
Cardizem
Cardoxin
Cardrase
Cardui
•carfecillin
carfentanil citrate
Cargesic
•carindacillin
Cari-Tab
carmantadine
Carmol HC
Carmol 20
carmustine
carnidazole
Caroid
caroxazone
•carperidine
carphenazine maleate
carprofen
cartazolate
carteolol hydrochloride
Cartose
Cartrax
carubicin hydrochloride
Casa-Dicole

Casafru
casanthranol
cascara sagrada
Casec
Casoate-A
Castaderm
Castel-Minus
Castellani Paint
castor oil
Casyllium
Catapres
Catarase
Causalin
Cavacaine
C-Bio
C-B-Plex
C-B Time
C-BE Zinc
C.D.M. Expectorant
Cea-Roche
Cebefortis
Cebenase
Cebetinic
Cebo-Caps
Cebral
Cebralan-M
Cebralan M.T.
Ceclor
Cecon
Cedilanid
Cedilanid-D
Ceeamide
Ceebevim
CeeNU
Ceepa
Ceepryn
Cee w/Bee Capsules
cefaclor

cefadroxil
Cefadyl
cefamandole
   c. nafate
   c. sodium
cefaparole
•cefapirin
cefatrizine
cefazaflur sodium
cefazolin sodium
Cefera
Cefinal II
Cefizox
cefmenoxime hydrochloride
Cefobid
Cefol Filmtabs
Cefomonil
cefonicid sodium
cefoperazone sodium
ceforanide
cefotaxime sodium
cefotiam hydrochloride
cefoxitin
   c. sodium
cefroxadine
cefsulodin sodium
ceftazidime
ceftizoxime sodium
ceftriaxone sodium
cefuroxime sodium
Celbenin
Celestone
Celestone Soluspan
celiprolol hydrochloride
•cellacephate
Cellepacbin
Cellothyl
Cellubolic

cellulase
cellulose, oxidized
Celoid
Celontin
Cel-U-Jec
Cemill
Cenabolic
Cenadex
Cenafed
Cenahist
Cenaid
Cena-K
Cenalax
Cenalene
Cenalone
CEN-E
Cenocort A-40
Cenocort Forte
Cenolate
Center-A1
Centrax
Centrine
Centrum
Centrum Jr.
Centuss
Ceo-Two
Cepacol
Cepastat
cephacetrile sodium
cephalexin
cephaloglycin
•cephalonium
•cephaloram
cephaloridine
cephalosporin
cephalothin sodium
cephapirin sodium
cephradine

Cephulac
Cerabex-T
Cerapon
Cerebel
Cerebid
Cerebro-Nicin
Cerespan
Cerose
Cerose-DM
Cerubidine
ceruletide diethylamine
Cerumenex
Cervex
Cervo
cesium chloride
cetaben sodium
Cetacaine
Cetacin
Cetacort
cetalkonium chloride
Cetamide
cetamolol hydrochloride
Cetane
Cetane-Caps TD
Cetaphil
Cetapred
Cetazol
cetiedil citrate
cetocycline hydrochloride
•cetomacrogol
cetophenicol
•cetoxime
cetraxate hydrochloride
Cetro-Cirose
cetylpyridinium chloride
Cevalin
Cevex
Cevi-Bid

Ce-Vi-Sol
Cevita
cevitamic acid:vitamin C
Cez
C.G.
C-G-10
CG RIA
Charcoaid
charcoal, activated
Charcocaps
Charcodote
Chardonna-2
Chek-Stix
Chel-Iron
Chemipen
Chemovag
Chenatal
Chenix
chenodiol
Cheque
Cheracol
Cheracol D
Cheracol Plus
Cheralin
Cherapas
Cherasulfa
Cheratussin
Cheri-Apro
Cherosed
Chero-Trisulfa-V
Cherralex
Cherri-B
Chestamine
Chew-Cee
Chew-E
Chew Hist
Chewies
Chew-Vims

Chew-Vi-Tab
Chew-Vite
Chexit
Chiggerex
Chigger-Tox
Children's Panadol
Chinosol
Chlo-Amine
chlophedianol hydrochloride
Chlor-4
Chlor-100
Chloracet
Chlorafed
Chlorafed Timecelles
Chlorahist
chloral betaine
    c. hydrate
Chloral-Methylol Ointment
Chloraman
Chloramate Unicelles
chlorambucil
chloramphenicol
    c. palmitate
    c. pantothenate complex
    c. sodium succinate
Chloraseptic
Chlor-A-Tyl
chlorazanil hydrochloride
chlorcyclizine hydrochloride
chlordantoin
chlordiazepoxide
    c. hydrochloride
Chloresium
Chloretone
chlorhexidine gluconate
    c. hydrochloride
Chlor-Hydro

Chlorhydrol
chlorindanol
chlorine
chloriodized oil
chlorisondamine chloride
chlormadinone acetate
Chlor-Mal
Chlormene
chlormerodrin Hg 197
    c. Hg 203
•chlormethiazole
chlormezanone
Chlor-Niramine
chloroazodin
chlorbutanol
Chlorocon
chlorocresol
chloroguanide hydrochloride
Chlorohist-LA
Chloromycetin
Chloromycetin Otic
Chloromyxin
Chlorophen
chlorophenothane
chlorophyll
chlorophyllin copper complex
chloroprocaine hydrochloride
Chloroptic
Chloroptic S.O.P.
Chloroptic-P S.O.P.
chloroquine
    c. hydrochloride
    c. phosphate
    c. sulfate
chlorothen citrate
chlorothiazide
    c. sodium
chlorotrianisene

chloroxine
chloroxylenol
Chlorphen
Chlorphenade
chlorphenesin carbamate
chlorpheniramine maleate
chlorphenoxamine
    hydrochloride
chlorphentermine
    hydrochloride
chlorproguanil
chlorpromazine
    hydrochloride
chlorpropamide
chlorprothixene
•chlorpyrifos
Chlor-PZ
•chlorquinaldol
Chlor-Rest
Chlor-Span
Chlorspan-12
Chlortab
chlortetracycline
    hydrochloride
chlorthalidone
Chlor-Trimeton
Chlortron
Chlorulan
Chlor-X
Chlorzide
Chlorzine
•chlorzoxazone
Cholan DH
Cholebrine
cholecalciferol
Choledyl
Choledyl SA
cholera vaccine

cholesterol
cholestyramine resin
Cholinate
choline bitartrate
    c. chloride
    c. dihydrogen citrate
    c. salicylate
Cho-Liv-12
Chol Meth in B
Cholografin
Cholografin Meglumine
Cholorebic
Cholovue
Choloxin
Cho-Meth
Choo E Plus C
Chooz
Chorex 5
Chorex 10
Chorigon
chorionic gonadotropin
Chorion-Plus
Choron
Christodyne-DHC
Chromagen
Chrometrace
chromic acid
    c. chloride
    c. chloride Cr 51
    c. phosphate Cr 51
    c. phosphate P 32
Chromitope Sodium
chromonar hydrochloride
Chronogyn
Chronulac
Chur-Hist
Chymar
Chymex

Chymodiactin
chymopapain
Chymoral
chymotrypsin
Cibalith-S
cibenzoline
ciclafrine hydrochloride
ciclopirox olamine
cicloprofen
Cidex
cimetidine
cinanserin hydrochloride
cinepazet maleate
•cinepazide
Cinex-40
cingestol
cinnamedrine
cinnarizine
Cinnasil
Cino-40
Cinobac
cinodine hydrochloride
Cinopal
cinoxacin
cinoxate
•cinoxolone
cinperene
Cin-Quin
cintazone
cintriamide
Cipralan
ciprefadol succinate
ciprocinonide
ciprofibrate
ciramadol
Ciramine
Cirbed
Circair

Circanol
Circavite-T
Circubid
Cirin
cirolemycin
cisplatin
citalopram
Citanest
citenamide
Cithal
Citra
Citra Forte
Citramin-500
Citrasan B
Citrasan K
Citrasan K-250
citrate
Citresco-K
citric acid
Citrobic
Citro-C
Citrocarbonate
Citrohist
Citrolith
Citro-Nesia
Citropam
Citrotein
C-Ject
CKA Canker Aid
Claforan
clamidoxic acid
clamoxyquin hydrochloride
clazolam
clazolimine
Clean-N-Soak
ClearAid
Clear & Brite
Clearasil

Clearasil BP
Clear by Design
CLD 2
Clear Eyes
Clearex
•clefamide
clemastine
      c. fumarate
•clenpyrin
Clens
Cleocin
      C. Pediatric
      C. Phosphate
      C. T
Clera
Clerz Drops
C-Lest
•cletoquine
clidinium bromide
clindamycin
      c. hydrochloride
      c. palmitate
         hydrochloride
      c. phosphate
Clindex
Clinicort
Clinicydin
Clinistix
Clinitest
Clinoril
Clinoxide
clioxanide
Clipoxide
cliprofen
Clistin
Clistin-D
Clistin RA
clocortolone acetate

clocortolone pivalate
Clocream
clodanolene
clodazon hydrochloride
Cloderm
clodronic acid
clofazimine
clofibrate
clofilium phosphate
cloflucarban
•clofluperol
clogestone acetate
•cloguanamil
clomacran phosphate
clomegestone acetate
clometherone
Clomid
clominorex
clomiphene citrate
clomipramine hydrochloride
•clomocycline
clonazepam
C-Long Granucaps
clonidine hydrochloride
•clonitazene
clonitrate
clonixeril
clonixin
Clonopin
clopamide
clopenthixol
cloperidone hydrochloride
clopidol
clopimozide
clopipazan mesylate
clopirac
•cloponone
cloprednol

cloprostenol sodium
•cloquinate
clorazepate dipotassium
     c. monopotassium
clorethate
clorexolone
Clorfed II
•clorgyline
•clorindione
cloroperone hydrochloride
clorophene
Clorpactin WCS-90
Clorpactin XCB
clorprenaline hydrochloride
clorsulon
clortermine hydrochloride
closantel
closiramine aceturate
clothiapine
clothixamide maleate
clotrimazole
Cloverine
Clovocain
cloxacillin
     c. sodium
Cloxapen
cloxyquin
clozapine
Clusivol 130
Clysodrast
Coactabs
Coactin
coal tar
Cobadoce Forte
cobalamin concentrate
Cobalasine
Cobalin
cobaltous chloride Co 57

cobaltous chloride Co 60
Coban
Cobatope-57
Cobatope-60
Cobefrin
Cobex 100
Co-Bile
Cobiron
cocaine
Cocillin V-K
Coco-Quinine
Codalan No. 1
Codalan No. 2
Codalex
Codamine
Codanol
Codap
Copaprin
Codasa I
Codasa II
Codasa Forte
Codehist DH
codeine
    c. phosphate
    c. sulfate
•co-dergocrine mesylate
Codiclear DH
Codimal
Codimal DH
Codimal DM
Codimal-L.A. Cenules
Codimal PH
Codistan No. 1
Coditrate
cod liver oil
codoxime
Codoxy
Codroxomin

Coenzyme-B
Co-Estro
Coffee Break
Co-Gel Liquitabs
Cogentin
Cohema
Co-Hep-Tral
Cohidrate
Co-Histine DH
Coidocort
Colace
Colagyn
Colana
•colaspase
Colate
Colax
ColBenemid
colchicine
Coldate
cold cream
Col-Decon
Coldonyl
Coldran
Coldrine
Colestid
colestipol hydrochloride
Col-Evac
Colexuss
Colfant
Colicell
colistimethate sodium
colistin sulfate
Colitussin
Co-Liver
Colladerm
collagenase
collodion
Collyrium

Coloctyl
Cologel
Colonatrast
Colonaid
Colrex
Colsalide
Coltab
colterol mesylate
Col-Vi-Nol
Coly-Mycin M
Coly-Mycin S
Coly-Mycin S Otic
Combantrin
Combex Kapseals
Combical D
Combichole
Combid
Combipres
Combistix
Combistrep
Comfolax
Comfolax-plus
Comfort Drops
Comfort Gel
Comfortine
Comhist
Comhist LA
Compazine
Compap
Compete
Compleat-B
Completabs
Compocillin-VK
Compound W
Compoz
Comprehensive Formula #28
Comprelets
Com-Pro-Span

Comtrex
Com-Vi-C
Comycin
Conacetol
Conalsyn
Conar
Conar-A
Conceptrol
Condecal
Condrin-LA
Conest
Conestoral
Conex
Conex D.A.
Conex Plus
Confident
Congespirin
Congess
Congess Sr.
Congest-Afed DM
Congesterone
Conhist
Co-Nib
Conjec
Conjugens
Conjutabs
Conray
Conray-30
Conray-400
Consin
Consotuss Antitussive
Constab-100
Constant-T
Constiban
Constonate 60
Contac
Contactisol
Contique

Contrapar
Controflex
Control
Controlyte
Converspaz
Converzyme
Cooper Creme
Copavin
Cope
Cophene
Cophene No. 2
Cophene-PL
Cophene-S
Cophene-X
Cophene-XP
Copin
Copperin
Coppertone
Coppertrace
Coprobate
Co-Pyronil
Co-Pyronil 2
Corace
Coracin
Coralsone
Coramine
Corane
Corbicin-125
Cordamine-PA
Cordilate
Cordran
Cordran-N
Cordran SP
Cordrol
Corega
Corgard
Corgonject-5
Coricidin

Coricidin D
Coricidin Demilets
Coricidin Medilets
Coriforte
Corilin
Corimist
Corlutin L.A.
cormethasone acetate
Corns-O-Poppin
Corodyl Forte
Cor-Oticin
Corovas Tymcaps
Corphos
Corque
Correctol
Corsym
Cortaid
Cortalone
Cortan
Cortane D.C.
Cortapp
Cortate
Cortcin
Cort-Dome
Cortef
Cortenema
Corticaine
Cortical
Corticoid
corticotropin (ACTH)
   c. zinc hydroxide
Cortifoam
Cortigel
Cortigesic
Cortikay
Cortin
Cortinal
Cortiprel

cortisone
   c. acetate
Cortisporin
Cortistan
cortivazol
Cortizone-5
Cort-Nib
cortodoxone
Cortogen
Cortone
Cort-Quin
Cortril
Cortril Acetate-AS
Cortrophin Gel
Cortrophin Zinc
Cortrosyn
Cort-Top
Corubeen
Corvaton
Coryban-D
Coryza Brengle Capsulets
Coryzaid
Coryzex
Coryztime
Corzans
Corzide
Corzone
Co-Sansprin
Cosanyl
Cosanyl-DM
Cosmegen
cosyntropin
Cotazym
Cotazym-B
Cotin
Co-Tinic
cotinine fumarate
Cotrim

Cotrim D.S.
•co-trimoxazole
Cotrol-D
Cotropic Gel 40
cotton, purified
Cotussis
CoTylenol
Cough EEZ
Coufarin
Coumadin
coumermycin
Counterpain
Covap
Covanamine
Covangesic
Covermark
Covicone
Co-Xan
CP
CP-2
C.P.C. Plus
CPI
Cplex
Creamalin
Cremagol
Cremesone
Creomulsin
Creosant
Creoterp
Creo-Terpin
Crescormon
cresol
Crestabolic
Cresylate
Criticare HN
Croferrin
crofilcon A
cromitrile sodium

cromolyn sodium
C-Ron
C-Ron Forte
C-Ron FA
•cropropamide
croscarmellose sodium
crotamiton
•crotethamide
crotoxyfos
Cruex
crufomate
Cryptocur
Cryspen-400
Crystallose
Crystamine
Crysticillin 300 A.S.
Crysticillin 600 A.S.
Crysti-Liver
Crystimin-1000
Crysti-12 Gel
Crysto-Gel
Crystodigin
Crystwel
C-Solve
C-Span
C Speridin
C-Syrup-500
CTD Complex
C-Tussin
Culminal
•cumetharol
Cuprex
cupric acetate
    c. chloride
    c. sulfate
Cuprimine
cuprimyxin
cuproxoline

Curatin
Curban
Curretab
Cutar
Cutemol
Cuticura
C.V.P.
Cyade-Gel
Cyamine
cyanide
Cyanocob
cyanocobalamin
    c. Co 57
    c. Co 60
Cyanoject
Cyanover
Cyantin
Cyasorb 5411
Cybis
cyclacillin
Cyclaine
cyclamic acid
Cyclapen-W
•cyclarbamate
cyclazocine
cyclindole
Cycline
cycliramine maleate
cyclizine
    c. hydrochloride
    c. lactate
cyclobarbital
•cyclobarbitone
Cyclo-Bell
cyclobendazole
cyclobenzaprine
  hydrochloride
Cyclocort

cyclocumarol
•cyclofenil
cyclofilcon A
Cyclogesterin
•cycloguanil embonate
cycloguanil pamoate
Cyclogyl
cycloheximide
cyclomethycaine sulfate
Cyclomine
Cyclomydril
Cyclopar
cyclopentamine
    hydrochloride
cyclopenthiazide
cyclopentolate hydrochloride
cyclophenazine hydrochloride
cyclophosphamide
cyclopropane
Cyclo-Prostin
cycloserine
Cyclospasmol
cyclosporine
Cyclo-Tab
cyclothiazide
cycrimine hydrochloride
Cydel
cyheptamide
Cylert
Cynobal

Cyomin
cypenamine hydrochloride
cyproheptadine
    hydrochloride
cyprolidol hydrochloride
cyproquinate
cyproterone acetate
cyproximide
Cystamine
cysteine hydrochloride
Cystex
cystine
Cystitol
Cysto
Cysto-Conray
Cystografin
Cystorelin
Cystosol
Cystospaz
Cystrea
Cytadren
cytarabine
    c. hydrochloride
Cytobolin
Cytoferin
Cytomel
Cytosar
Cytosar-U
Cytoxan
Cyvaso

D

dacarbazine
Dacriose
Dactil
dactinomycin
dacuronium bromide
Dagenan
Daily/Jet
Daily Vite
Dainite
Dainite-KI
Dalalone
Dalalone D.P.
Dalalone I.L.
Dalalone L.A.
Dalaron
Dalaron L.A.
Dalca
Dalcaine
daledalin tosylate
Dalfatol
Dalgan
Dalicote
Dalicreme
Daliderm
Dalidyne
Dalifort
Daligesic
Dalihist
Dalimycin
Dalisept
Dalivim Forte
Dallergy
Dalmane

Dalnate
D-Alpha-E Cap
Damason-P
D-Amp
danazol
Danex
Danivac
Danker Silicone Lens
Danocrine
Dantafur
Danthane
danthron
Danthross
Dantrium
dantrolene
   d. sodium
Danvac
Dapa
Dapco
dapsone
Dap-Test Macro
Daragen
Daranide
Daraprim
Darbid
Darcil
Darco G-60
Daricon
Daricon-PB
Darifur
Daro Tablets-C.T.
Dartal
Darvocet-N

Darvon
Darvon-N
Darvon with A.S.A.
Da-Sed
Dasikon
Dasin
D-Asma-S
Datril
Datril 500
Daturine HBr
daunorubicin hydrochloride
Davisol
Daxid
Dayalets
Day Caps
DayCare
Day-Tabs
Day-Vite
dazadrol maleate
dazoxiben hydrochloride
D-Caine
DCP
DDAVP
D-Diol
Deaner
Deapril-ST
Debrisan
debrisoquin sulfate
Debrox
Decaderm
Decadron
Decadron-LA
Deca-Durabolin
Decaject
Decaject LA
De-Cal
Decalix
Decameth L.A.

decamethonium bromide
Decapryn
Decaspray
Deca-Vi-Sol
Deccasol-T
Decholin
declenperone
Declinax
Declomycin
Declostatin
Decobel
Decohist
Decojen
Decolone-50
De-Comberol
Deconade
Deconamine
Deconex
Decontabs
decoquinate
dectaflur
Decubitex
Decuritis
Deep-Down Rub
deferoxamine
  d. hydrochloride
  d. mesylate
•defibrotide
Deficol
d-Film
Definate
Degest
Dehist
dehydrocholate sodium
dehydrocholic acid
•dehydroemetine
Deka
Deka-Vites

Delacort
Deladiol-40
Deladumone
Deladumone OB
Delalutin
Delanex
Del-Anthra
Delapav
Delaquin
Delatest
Delatestadiol
Delatestryl
Delaxin
Delcid
Del-Clens
Del-Trac
Del-Stat
Delcobese
Delco-Lax
Delcoplex
Delco-Retic
Delcozine
Delcronol
Delestrec
Delestrogen
Delfen
Delladec
delmadinone acetate
Delmate
Delsym Pennkinetic
Delta-Cortef
Delta-E
deltafilcon A
Deltalin
Deltalin Gelseals
Deltamycin
Deltapen-VK
Deltasone

Deltavac
Deltoin
Deltra
Deluteval
Delvinal
Demasone-LA
Demazin
demecarium bromide
demeclocycline
    d. hydrochloride
•demecolcine
demecycline
Demerol
Demi-Regroton
demoxepam
Demser
Demulen
Demulen 1/35-21
Demure
denatonium benzoate
Dencorub
Dendrid
Dengesic
denofungin
Denorex
Denquel
Dentavite
Dentofluor Drops
Dentoid
Denylex Gel
•deoxycortone acetate
D.E.P.-75
Depakene
Depakote
Depanate
depAndro 100
depAndrogyn
Depapred IP

depCorlutin
Depen Titratabs
Depepsen
Dep-Estradiol
Depestro
depGynogen
Depinar
Depletite
depMedalone 40
depMedalone 80
Depogen
Depo-Acth
Depo-Medrol
Depo-Pred
Depo-Provera
Depotest
Depo-Testadiol
Depotestogen
Depo-Testosterone
depPredalone
Deproist
Deprol
Deprolutin-250
deprostil
Dep-Test
Dep-Testosterone
Dep-Testradiol
•deptropine
•dequalinium chloride
DEQUAsine
Dequibolin-l00
Derfule
Derifil
Derisol
Dermacare
Dermacon
Dermacort
Derma-Cover

Derma-Guard
Derm-Aid
Dermal-Rub
Derma Medicone
Derma Medicone-HC
Dermamycin
Derma-Pax
Dermaphill
Derma-pH
Dermarex
Derma-Smoothe/FS
Derma-Sone
Dermassage
Derma Soap
Derma-Soft
Dermasorcin
Dermastringe
Dermasul
Dermathyn
Dermatophytin O
Dermax
Dermeze
DermiCort
Dermidon
Dermolate
Dermolin
Dermoplast
Dermovan
Dermtex
Deronil
Desacholine
Desa-Hist AT
Desa-Hist PF
Desamycin
descinolone acetonide
Desenex
De Serpa
Desferal

desipramine hydrochloride
Desitin
deslanoside
Desma
desmopressin acetate
Deso-Creme
•desomorphine
desonide
desoximetasone
desoxycorticosterone acetate
  d. pivalate
  d. trimethylacetate
Desoxyn
desoxyribonuclease
Desquam-X
D-Est
Desyrel
Detachol
De Tal
Detane
deterenol hydrochloride
DeTone 0.1
Detrothyronine
De-Tuss
Detussin
deuterium oxide
Devegan
Devine's Kool Foot
Devrom
Devryl
Dex-A-Cel
Dexacen-4
Dexacen LA-8
dexamethasone
  d. acetate
  d. sodium phosphate
dexamisole
Dexampex

•dexamphetamine
Dexaport
Dexasone
Dexasone-LA
Dexatrim
dexbrompheniramine
  maleate
Dexbrom T.D.
dexchlorpheniramine maleate
dexclamol hydrochloride
Dexedrine
dexetimide
deximafen
dexivacaine
Dexon
Dexon LA
Dexone
Dexone LA
Dexone TM
Dexoval
dexoxadrol hydrochloride
dexpanthenol
dexpropranolol hydrochloride
Dex-Salt
Dexone
dextran 40
dextran 70
dextran 75
•dextranomer
dextrates
dextroamphetamine
  d. phosphate
  d. sulfate
Dextrobar
Dextrocaine
Dextrocell
Dextromal
dextromethorphan

dextromethorphan
  (*continued*)
    d. hydrobromide
• dextropropoxyphene
  hydrochloride
• dextrorphan
dextrose
Dextrostix
dextrothyroxine sodium
Dextro-Tuss GG
Dexule
Dexyl
Dexzone
Dexzone LA
Dey-Dose
Dey-Sol
dezocine
Dezone
D-Film
D.H.E.45
DHT
Diabeta
Diabetussin
Diabinese
Diabismul
• diacetamate
Diaceto
diacetolol hydrochloride
diacetylmorphine
  hydrochloride
Diacin
Diaction
Diadax
Di-Ademil
Diadol
Dia-Eze
Diafen
Diahist

Dial
Dialixir
Dialog
Dialose
Dialume
diamocaine cyclamate
Diamox
• diampromide
Dianabol
Dianeal
Dianeal 137
Dianeal K
Dianeal K-141
Diapa-Kare
diapamide
Diaparene
Diapid
Diaparess
Di-Ap-Trol
Diaqua
Dia-Quel
Diar-Aid
Diarcon
Diarkote
Diarrest
Diasone
Diasporal
Diastay
Diastix
Diastix 5
Diatric
diatrizoate meglumine
    d. sodium
    d. sodium I 125
    d. sodium I 131
diatrizoic acid
diaveridine
diazepam

•diazinon
diaziquone
Di-Azo
diazoxide
•dibekacin
Dibenamine
Dibent
Dibent-PB
dibenzepin hydrochloride
Dibenzyline
Dibestil
dibromsalan
dibucaine
    d. hydrochloride
Dibuline
•dibupyrone
dibutoline sulfate
Dical-Caps
Dical-D
Dical-Dee
Dicaldel
Dicaltabs
Dicarbosil
Dicen
Di-Cet
•dichlofenthion
dichlorotetrafluoroethane
•dichloroxylenol
dichlorphenamide
dichlorvos
Dicholin
diclofenac sodium
dicloralurea
dicloxacillin
    d. sodium
Dicloxin
Dicodid
Dicodrine

Dicole
•dicophane
Dicotrate
dicumarol
Dicurin Procaine
dicyclomine hydrochloride
Di-Cyclonex
Dicyclon-M
Dicyclon No. 1, No. 2, No. 3
Di-Delamine
Didrate
Didrex
Didronel
•dieldrin
dienestrol
Dietac
Dietene
Diet-Gard
•diethadione
diethylcarbamazine citrate
diethyl phthalate
diethylpropion hydrochloride
diethylstilbestrol: DES
    d. diphosphate
•diethylthiambutene
diethyltoluamide
Diet Plan
Diet-Trim
Diet-Tuss
Di-Factor
difenoximide hydrochloride
difenoxin
•difetarsone
diflorasone diacetate
difluanine hydrochloride
diflucortolone
    d. pivalate
diflumidone sodium

diflunisal
difluprednate
diftalone
Di-Gel
Digenzymes
Di-Gesic
Digesplen
Digestalin
Digestamic
Digestant
Digestex
Digifortis Kapseals
Digiglusin
Digitaline Nativelle
digitalis
digitoxin
Digolase
digoxin
dihexyverine hydrochloride
Dihistine
Dihycon
Dihydrex
dihydroergotamine mesylate
dihydrotachysterol
dihydroxyaluminum
  aminoacetate
    d. sodium carbonate
dihydroxypropyl theophylline
diisopropanolamine
Dilabil
Dilacap
Dilantin
Dilart
Dilart-300
Dilatrate Sr.
Dilaudid
Dilaudid-HP
Dilax

Dilin
Dilocaine
Dilocol
Dilomine
Dilone
Dilor
Dilor 400
Dilorex
Dilor G
•diloxanide
diltiazem hydrochloride
Dimacid
Dimacol
Dimalix
Dimate
dimefadane
dimefilcon A
dimefline hydrochloride
dimefocon A
dimenhydrinate
•dimenoxadol
Dimentabs
•dimepheptanol
•dimepregnen
•dimepropion
dimercaprol
•dimesone
Dimetane
Dimetane-Ten
Dimetapp
dimethadione
dimethicone
dimethicone 350
dimethindene maleate
dimethisoquin hydrochloride
dimethisterone
dimethoxanate hydrochloride
dimethothiazine

dimethyl sulfoxide: DMSO
•dimetridazole
diminazene
Dimindol
Dimocillin
dimoxamine hydrochloride
Dimycor
Dinacrin
Dinate
•dinitolmide
dinoprost
    d. tromethamine
dinoprostone
dinsed
Dioctin
Diocto
Diodone
Diodoquin
Diodrast
Dioeze
Diogyn
Diogyn E
Diogynets
diohippuric acid I-125
    d. acid I-131
Dio-Hist
Diolax
DioMedicone
Dionex
Dionosil
Diorapin
Diostate D
Diosuccin
Dio-Sul
Diosux
Diothane
Diothron
diotyrosine I-125

diotyrosine I-131
Dioval
Dioval XX
Dioval 40
dioxadrol hydrochloride
•dioxaphetyl butyrate
Dioxatrine
dioxybenzone
dioxyline phosphate
Dipav
Dipaxin
dipendrate
•dipenine bromide
diperodon
diphemanil methylsulfate
Di-Phen
diphenadione
Diphenadril
Diphenatol
Diphen-Ex
diphenhydramine
    hydrochloride
diphenidol
    d. hydrochloride
    d. pamoate
diphenoxylate hydrochloride
diphenylpyraline
    hydrochloride
diphtheria antitoxin
Diphylets
Diphylets-T
•dipipanone
dipivefrin
Diplan
Di-Pred
•diprenorphine
•diprobutine
Diprolene

•diprophylline
Diprosone
dipyridamole
dipyrithione
dipyrone
Dirame
Diridone
Disalcid
Disanthrol
Discase
Disipal
Dismiss
disobutamide
disofenin
Disolan
Disolan Forte
Disonate
Disophrol
disopyramide
    d. phosphate
Di-Sosul
Di-Sosul Forte
Diso-Tate
Di-Spaz
Dispos-a-Med
Disulans
Disulans-Plus
disulfiram
Ditan
Ditate
Ditate-DS
D.I.T.I. Creme
D.I.T.I.-2 Creme
Ditropan
Diucardin
Diulo
Diupres
Diurese

Diurese-R
Diuretane #1, #2
Diuretin
Diuril
Diu-Scrip
Diu-Tabs
Diutensen
Diutensen-R
divalproex sodium
Divarine
Divaso
Diviron
Dizmiss
D-Med-80
DMSO: dimethyl sulfoxide
DNR: daunorubicin
Doak-Oil
Doan's Rub
Dobell's Solution
dobutamine
    d. hydrochloride
Dobutrex
Doca Acetate
doconazole
Doctate 100
Doctate 300
Doctate-P
Doctient HC
Doctyl
Doctylax
docusate calcium
    d. potassium
    d. sodium
Dodamin
Dodex
•dofamium chloride
DoFus
doktors nose drops

Dolacet
Dolamin
Dolanex
Dolcin
Doldram
Dolear
Dolene
Dolene AP-65
Dolex
Dolicaine
Dolobid
Dolomite
Dolonil
Dolopar
Dolophine
Doloral
Dolorgon
Dolsed
domazoline fumarate
Domeboro
Domeform-HC
Dome-Paste
Domerine
domiodol
domiphen bromide
Dommanate
domperidone
Donabarb
Donatussin
Dondril
Donna
Donnacin
Donnafed Jr.
Donnagel
Donnagel-PG
Donnamine
Donnamor
Donna-Phenal

Donnaphen
Donna-Sed
Donnatal
Donnazyme
Donphen
dopamantine
dopamine hydrochloride
Dopar
Dopastat
Dophenco
Dopram
Dorantamin
Doraphen Compound 65
dorastine hydrochloride
Dorbane
Dorbantyl
Dorbantyl Forte
Dorcol
Doriden
Dorimide
Dormarex
Dormate
Dorme
Dormeer
Dormethan
Dormin
Dormutol
Dorsacaine
Dorsital
Doss 300
dothiepin hydrochloride
Dovamide
Dovaphen
Doveram
Dovium
Dow-Isoniazid
Doxamin
Doxan

doxapram hydrochloride
doxaprost
doxazosin mesylate
doxepin hydrochloride
Doxidan
Doxinate
doxorubicin
    d. hydrochloride
doxpicomine hydrochloride
Doxy-C
doxycycline
    d. calcium
    d. hyclate
doxylamine succinate
Doxy-Lemmon
Doxy-Tabs
Doxy-II
Dralserp
Dralzine
Dramaban
Dramal
Dramamine
Dramilin
Dramocen
Dranochol
Dramoject
Drest
Dri-Drip
Dri-A Caps
Dri A & D Caps
Dri-E
Dri/Ear
Dri-Hist Meta-Kaps
Drinalfa
drinidene
Drinophen
Drinus
Drinus-M

Drisdol
Dristan
Dristan-AF
Drithocreme
Drixoral
Drize
drobuline
drocinonide
Drolban
drometrizole
dromostanolone propionate
Droncit
droperidol
dropropizine
•drotebanol
Drotic
droxacin sodium
droxifilcon A
Droxine L.A.
Droxine S.F.
Droxolan
Droxomin
Droxovite
•droxypropine
Drucon
Dry and Clear
Drysol
Drysum
Drytergent
Drytex
Dryvax
D-seb Gel
D-Sinus
D-S-S Capsules
D-Test 200
DTIC-Dome
Duadacin
Dualex-E

Dua-Pred
duazomycin
Ducobee-Hy
Dulcolax
Du-Min
Duo-Cyp
Duofilm
Duo-FLow
Duogen L.A. 90/4
Duo-Gen L.A. 180/8
Duo-Hist
Duo-Ionate
Duoject
Duo-K
Duolip
Duolube
Duo-Medihaler
Duomine
Duoprin
Duoprin-S
Duo-strep
Duosorb
Duosol
Duotal
Duo-Trach Kit
Duotrate
Duotrate-45
Duotrone
Duoval-PA
Duovent
Duovin-S
Duo-WR, No. 1, No. 2
Duphalac
Duphrene
Duphaston
Duphrene
Duplast
Duplex T

Dura-12-M
Durabolic
Durabolin
Durabolin-50
Dura-C 500
Dura-Chorion
Duracillin
Duradyne
Duradyne DHC
Duradyne Forte
Dura-Estrin
Duragen
Duragesic
Dura-Kellin
Duralex
Duralone
Dura-Meth
Duramid
Duramist
Durandrol
Duranest
Duranest HCl
durapatite
Durapav
Duraphyl
Durapred
Durapred T.B.A.
Duraquin
Durasal
Durasil
DuraSoft
Duratears
Duratest
Durathesia
Duration
Dura-Vent
Durrax
Durel-Cort

Durel-Cort 'V'
Dureze Otic Drops
Duricef
Duvoid
D-Vaso
D-Vaso-S
Dwiatol
Dyazide
Dycill
Dyclone
dyclonine hydrochloride
Dycolate
Dycomene
dydrogesterone
Dyflex
Dyflex-G

•dyflos
Dyline-GG
Dymelor
Dymenate
Dynamutilin
Dynamyxin
Dynapen
Dynohist S.A.
Dynosal
Dy-O-Derm
dyphylline
Dyrenium
Dyrexam-O.D.
Dysenaid Jr.
Dyspel

E

Earcaine
Eardro
Ear-Dry
Earex
Ear-Ol
Easprin
East-A
East-Gesic
Eastinic
East-Nata
East-Serpine
Easy-Lax
Eazol
E-Carpine
Ecee Plus
Echodide
echothiophate iodide

Eclabron
Eclipse After Sun Lotion
Ecodide
Ecofrol
econazole
    e. nitrate
Econo B & C Capsules
Econochlor
Econopred
Ecostatin
Ecotrin
E Cream
Ectasule III
Ectol
Edecrin
edetate calcium disodium
    e. dipotassium

edetate (*continued*)
   e. disodium
   e. sodium
   e. trisodium
edetol
•edogestrone
Edrised
edrophonium
  chloride
E-Dust
E.E.S.
Efed
Efed II
Efedra P.A.
Efedron Nasal
E-Ferol
E-Ferol Succinate
Efficin
Efodine
Efricel
Efricon
Efudex
Ego
egtazic acid
E-Ionate P.A.
elantrine
Elaqua XX
Elase
elastofilcon A
Elastoplast
Elavil
Eldadryl
El-Da-Mint
Eldatapp
Eldec
Eldecort
Eldekal
Elder 65

Eldercaps
Eldertonic Elixir
Eldisine
Eldo-B & C
Eldodram
Eldofe
Eldofe-C
Eldonal
Eldopaque
Eldoquin
Eldothane
Eldovite
Elecal
Elegen-G
Elekap
elfazepam
Elite
Elipten
Elixicon
Elixiral
Elixomin
Elixophyllin
Elixophyllin-GG
Elixophyllin-KI
Elixophyllin SR
Elixsed
Ellesdine
Elmotil
Eloxyl
EL-PETN
Elphemet
Elprecal
Elserpine
Elspar
elucaine
Elvanol
Elzyme
Emagrin

Emagrin Forte
embramine
embutramide
Emcol E-607
EMCYT
Emdol
•emepronium bromide
Emeroid
Emerest 2355
Emersal
Emesis
Emete-Con
Emeticon
emetine hydrochloride
Emetrol
Emfabid
Emfaseem
emilium tosylate
Emko
Emko Pre-Fil
Empirin
Empracet
Emprazil
Emprazil-C
Emtryl
Emtrymix
Emulave
Emul-O-Balm
Emulsoil
E-Mycin
E-Mycin E
enalapril maleate
Enarax
E-Natural
•enbucrilate
encainide hydrochloride
Encare
En-Cebrin

En-Cebrin F
enclomiphene
encyprate
End-Ake
Endal
Endecon
Endep
End-Itch
Endotussin-NN
Endoxan
endralazine mesylate
Endrate
endrysone
Enduron
Enduronyl
Enduronyl Forte
Energetts
Enfamil
enflurane
Engran-HP
enilconazole
Enisyl
Enkade
Ennex
ENO
enolicam sodium
Enovid
Enovid-E 21
Enovil
Enoxa
•enoxolone
enpromate
Enrumay
Ensure
Ensure Plus
E.N.T.
Entab-650
Entericin

Entero-Vioform
Entex
Entex L.A.
Entodon
Entozyme
entsufon sodium
Entuss
Enuclene
Enuretrol
Envacar
enviradene
enviroxime
Enzactin
Enzeon
Enzest
Enzobile
Enzopride
Enzymet
Enzypan
ephedrine
    e. hydrochloride
    e. sulfate
Ephedsol-1
Ephenyllin
Ephrine
Ephrinite No.1
Epicar
epicillin
Epicort
Epifoam
Epiform-HC
Epifrin
E-Pilo
epimestrol
Epimorph
Epimycin A
Epinal
Epinephricaine

epinephrine
    e. bitartrate
epinephryl borate
EpiPen Jr.
epipropidine
epirizole
Episone
epithiazide
Epitrate
E-Plus
Eponal
Eponal-G
epoprostenol
    e. sodium
Eprolin
Epsal
Epsilan-M
Epsivite Forte
epsom salt
Equagesic
Equagesic-M
Equal
Equanil
Equanitrate
Equiben
Equibolin-50
Equigard
Equigel
Equilet
equilin
Equine-Atom Elixir
Equizole
Eramycin
Erasen
Ercaf
Ercal
Ercatab
Ergamisol

Ergobel
Ergo-Caff
ergocalciferol
Ergomar
ergoloid mesylates
ergonovine
   e. maleate
Ergophene
Ergostat
ergotamine tartrate
Ergotrate Maleate
Ergozide
Eridione
E-R-O Drops
ERO Forte Otic
Ertine
Ertron
EryDerm
Erymax
Erypar
EryPed
Ery-Tab
erythrityl tetranitrate
Erythrocin
Erythrocin Lactobionate-IV
Erythrocin Stearate
erythromycin
   e. estolate
   e. ethylsuccinate
   e. gluceptate
   e. lactobionate
   e. propionate
   e. stearate
erythrosine sodium
Escot
Esdone
Esgic
Esidrix

Esimil
Eskalith
E-Solve
Esophotrast
Esorb
Esoterica
Especol
Espotabs
E.S.P.R.
esproquin hydrochloride
Estaqua
Estar
Estate
Estercol
Estergel
esterifilcon A
Esterigyn
Estinyl
Estivin
Estomul-M
Estra-C
Estra-V
Estrace
estradiol
   e. benzoate
   e. enanthate
   e. undecylate
   e. valerate
Estradurin
Estraguard
Estra-L 20
estramustine
   e. phosphate sodium
Estran-C
Estran-E.V.
Estratab
Estratest
Estratest H.S.

Estra-Testrin
Estraval
Estraval PA
Estraval 2X
Estra-Vate
estrazinol hydrobromide
estriol
Estritone No.1, No.2
Estroate
Estro-Cyp
Estrofem
Estrofol
estrofurate
Estroject
Estroject-L.A.
Estrol
estrone
Estronol
estropipate
Estro Plus
Estroquin
Estrovis
Estrusol
etafedrine hydrochloride
etafilcon A
•etamiphyllin
etazolate hydrochloride
•etenzamide
eterobarb
ethacrynate sodium
ethacrynic acid
ethambutol hydrochloride
ethamivan
ethamsylate
ethanol
Ethaquin
Ethatab
Ethav

ethchlorvynol
ether
ethinamate
ethinyl estradiol
ethiodized oil I-131
Ethiodol
Ethiodol-131
ethiofos
ethionamide
ethohexadiol
•ethomoxane
ethonam nitrate
ethopropazine hydrochloride
ethosuximide
ethoxazene hydrochloride
ethoxzolamide
Ethrane
Ethril
ethybenztropine
ethyl acetate
    e. alcohol
    e. chloride
    e. dibunate
    e. ether
ethylene
ethylenediamine
ethylestrenol
ethylnorepinephrine
   hydrochloride
ethylparaben
ethynerone
ethynodiol diacetate
etibendazole
etidocaine hydrochloride
etidronate disodium
etidronic acid
etifenin
etintidine hydrochloride

etodolac
etoformin hydrochloride
etomidate
etoposide
etoprine
•etorphine
etoxadrol hydrochloride
etozolin
Etrafon
Etrenol
etretinate
Etrynit
etryptamine acetate
eucatropine hydrochloride
Eucerin
Eugel
eugenol
Eulcin
Eumydrin
Euphenex
Euphorbia Compound
euprocin hydrochloride
Eurax
Euresol
Euthroid
Eutonyl
Eutron Filmtabs
Evac-Q-Kit
Evac-Q-Kwik
Evac-Q-Mag
Evac-Q-Tabs
Evactol
Evac-U-Gen
Evac-U-Lax
evans blue

Evenol 400
Everone
Evestrone
Evex
Evipal
Eviron
Eviron FA
Eviron FT
E-Vista
E-Vitabon
E-Vital
E-Vites
Ex-Apap
exaprolol hydrochloride
Ex-Aqua
Excedrin
Excedrin P.M.
Ex-Lax
Exna
Exocaine
Exo-Kol
Expansatol
Expectrosed
Exsel
Extend
Extend l2
Extendac
Extendryl Sr.
Extralin
Exul
Exzit
Eye-Cort
Eye-Gene
Eye-Sed
Eye-Stream

F

Factorate
Fact Pregnancy Kit
Factrel
Falmonox
famotine hydrochloride
Fanasil
fanetizole mesylate
Fansidar
fantridone hydrochloride
Fara-Gel
Fara-Sin
Faratac
Faratol
Faratuss
Fasigyn
Fastin
FBC
F.C.A.H.
febantel
Feberin
Febrigesic
Febrinol
Fe-Brone
Fecoplex
Feco-T
Fedahist
Fedahist Gyrocaps
Fedrazil
Fedrelen
Fedrex
Fedrinal
Feen-a-Mint
Feldene

Fellozine
Felsules
felypressin
Femagene
Femcaps
Femeze
Femguard
Fem-H
Femidine
Feminate-10
Feminins
Feminone
Femogen
Femogen-L.A.
Femotrone
Femspan
fenalamide
fenamole
fenbendazole
fenbufen
Fenbutal
•fencamfamin
fencibutirol
fenclofenac
fenclonine
fenclorac
•fenclozic acid
Fendol
fendosal
fenestrel
fenethylline hydrochloride
fenfluramine hydrochloride
fenimide

fenisorex
fenmetozole hydrochloride
fenobam
fenoctimine sulfate
fenoprofen
   f. calcium
fenoterol
fenpipalone
•fenpiprane
fenprinast hydrochloride
fenprostalene
fenquizone
fenspiride hydrochloride
fentanyl citrate
fenticlor
fenticonazole nitrate
Fenylhist
Fenylex
fenyripol hydrochloride
Feocyte
Feosol
Feostat
Feostim
F-E-P
Fe-Plus
•feprazone
Ferancee
Ferancee-HP
Ferate-C
Feratin
Fergon
Fer-In-Sol
Fermalox
Ferndex
Fernhist
Fernisolone-P
Fernisone
Ferocyl

Fero-Folic-500
Fero-Gradumet
Fero-Grad-500 Filmtabs
Ferolate
Ferolix
Feronate
Ferospace
Ferotran
Ferotrinsic
Ferracomp
Ferradoss
Ferralet
Ferralyn Lanacaps
Ferranol
Ferric-B Jr.
ferric chloride Fe 59
ferric fructose
ferriclate calcium sodium
Ferrinal-C
Ferrinal Chroncap
Ferrobid
Ferro-Chek II
Ferro-Cyte
Ferrolip
Ferroneed
Ferronese
Ferronex
Ferro Plus
Ferro-Sequels
Ferrospan
Ferrosyn
Ferrosyn S.C.
ferrous citrate Fe 59
ferrous fumarate
Ferrous-G
ferrous gluconate
ferrous sulfate
ferrous sulfate Fe 59

Ferusal
Fesotyme
Festal
Festalan
Festex
fetoxylate hydrochloride
Fibocil
fibrinogen I 125
Filibon
Filibon F.A.
Filibon Forte
Filibon OT
filipin
Filtrosol A
Finac
Fiogesic
Fiorinal
Firmdent
Fixodent
Fizrin
Flacid
Flagyl
Flagyl I.V.
Flatus
Flav-A-D
Flavihist
flavodilol maleate
Flavomycin
Flavorcee
flavoxate hydrochloride
Flaxedil
flazalone
flecainide acetate
Fleet Bagenema
Fleet Barobag
Fleet Bisacodyl
Fleet enema
Fleet Relief

Flenac
fletazepam
Flexaphen
Flex-Care
Flexeril
Flexoject
Flexon
Flexsol 43
Flo-Cillin
floctafenine
Florajen
•florantyrone
Flor-D
flordipine
Florical
Floridin
Florinef
Florital
Florone
Floropryl
Florvite
floxacillin
Floxapen
floxuridine
•fluanisone
Fluax
fluazacort
flubanilate hydrochloride
flubendazole
flucindole
flucloronide
Flucort
flucrylate
flucytosine
fludalanine
fludarabine phosphate
fludazonium chloride
fludorex

fludrocortisone acetate
flufenamic acid
flufenisal
Fluidex Plus
Fluidil
Flu-Immune
•flumedroxone
flumequine
flumeridone
flumethasone
    f. pivalate
•flumethiazide
•flumethrin
flumetramide
flumezapine
fluminorex
flumizole
flumoxonide
flunarizine hydrochloride
flunidazole
flunisolide
flunitrazepam
flunixin
fluocinolone acetonide
fluocinonide
fluocortin butyl
fluocortolone
    f. caproate
Fluogen
Fluonid
•fluopromazine
Fluoral
fluorescein
    f. sodium
Fluorescite
Fluoreseptic
Fluoresoft
Fluorigard

Fluorineed
Fluorinse
Fluor-I-Strip
Fluoritab
fluorometholone
Fluoroplex
fluorosalan
Fluoroseptic
fluorouracil
Fluothane
fluotracen hydrochloride
fluoxetine
fluoxymesterone
fluperamide
fluperolone acetate
fluphenazine enanthate
    f. hydrochloride
fluprednisolone
    f. valerate
fluprofen
fluproquazone
fluprostenol sodium
fluquazone
Flura
Flura-Drops
Flura-Loz
flurandrenolide
•flurandrenolone
Flura-Pren
Flura-Vite
flurazepam hydrochloride
flurbiprofen
Fluress
fluretofen
flurocitabine
flurofamide
flurogestone acetate
Flurosyn

flurothyl
fluroxene
fluspiperone
fluspirilene
flutamide
Flutex
flutiazin
Fluzone-Connaught
F.M.-400
FML Liquifilm
Foille
Folabee
Folex
folic acid
Folicet
Fol-Li-Bee Forte
Follutein
Folvite
Folvron
Fomac
fonazine mesylate
Forane
Forbutol
Forhistal Maleate
Forit
formaldehyde
•formebolone
•forminitrazole
formocortal
Formula 44
Formula-75
Formula 405
Forte L.I.V.
Fortespan
Forthane
fosazepam
fosfomycin
fosfonet sodium

Fosfree
fospirate
Fostex
Fostex BPO
Fostex CM
Fostex 10
Fostril
4-Way Cold Tablets
4-Way Nasal Spray
Four Red
Foursalco
Fowler's Solution
Foygen
Foyuretic
•framycetin
FreAmine II
Freezone
Frepp
Frepp/Sepp
fructose
Fuadin
fuchsin
Ful-Glo
Fulvicin-P/G
Fulvicin-U/F
•fumagillin
Fumasorb
Fumatinic
Fumatrin-Forte
Fumerin
Fumidil
Fumiron
Funduscein
Fungacetin
fungimycin
Fungizone
Fungoid
Fung-o-Spray

Fungotic
Furacin
Furacort
furacrinic acid
Furadantin
Furadex
Furalan
Furamazone
Furan
furaprofen
Furaspor
furazolidone
furazolium chloride
    f. tartrate

Furea
•furethidine
furobufen
furodazole
furosemide
Furox
Furoxone
fursalan
•fusafungine
fusidate sodium
fusidic acid
Fusinol

G

G-1
G-2
G-3
G-11
G-200
gallamine triethiodide
gallium citrate Ga 67
Gamastan
gamfexine
Gamimune
Gammagee
Gammar
Ganatrex
Ganphen
Gantanol
Gantrex

Gantrisin
Garamycin
Garitabs
Garrathion
Gasticans
Gastrical
Gastrografin
Gastrovist
Gas-X
Gaviscon
Gaviscon-2
Gaysal-S
G.B.S.
Gel Clean
Gelfilm
Gelflex

Gelfoam
Gel-Kam
Gelocast
Gelpirin
Gelsaf
Geltabs
Gel-Tin
Gelusil
Gelusil-M
Gelusil-II
gemcadiol
gemeprost
gemfibrozil
Gemnisyn
Gemonil
Genabol
Genapax
Genoptic
gentamicin sulfate
gentian violet
Gentlax S
Gentran
Gentran 40
Gentran 75
Gentz
Geocillin
Geopen
Gera-B
Geralix
Geravite
Geriamic
Geriatrazole
Geriatro-B
Geriatroplex
Geriban
Geribom
Geriden
Gerifort

Gerigard
Gerijen
Gerilets
Geriliquid
Gerilite Elixir
Gerimal
Gerinats-H
Gerinats-T
Gerineed
Geripan
Geriplex-FS
Geri-Plus
Gerisol
Gerispan
Geritag
Geritinic
Geritol
Geritol Mega Vitamins
Geritonic
Gerivites
Gerix Elixir
Gerizyme
Gerlipo
Germa-Medica
Germicin
Germ-i-Tol
Ger-O-Foam
Geroniazol TT
Gerovital H3
Gerren
Gesic
gestaclone
Gesterol 100
Gesterol L.A. 250
Gest
gestonorone caproate
gestrinone
• gestronol

Gets-It Liquid
Gevrabon
Gevral
Gevral T
Gevrite
GG-CEN
G.G.I.
G.G.-Tussin
Ginsocap
Gispasmin
Gitaligin
Glaucon
Glaucostat
gleptoferron
gliamilide
• glibenclamide
Glibenese
glibornuride
glicetanile sodium
• gliclazide
gliflumide
glipizide
• gliquidone
• glisoxepide
globulin, immune serum
gloxazone
glucagon
gluceptate sodium
Gluco-Ferrum
Glucola
glucosamine
Glucoron
Glucovite
Glu-K
Glukor
glutaral
Glutest
glutethimide

Glutofac
Glutol
Glutose
glyburide
• glycalox
Glycate
glycerin
Glyceryl-T
• glyceryl trinitrate
glycobiarsol
glycol distearate
glycopyrrolate
• glycopyrronium bromide
Glycotuss
Glycotuss-dM
• glycyclamide
Glydeine
glymidine sodium
Glynazan
glyoctamide
Gly-Oxide
glyparamide
Glyrol
Glysennid
Glytabs
Glytinic
Gly-Trate
Glytuss
Glyvenol
gold Au l98
gold sodium thiomalate
Gonadex
gonadorelin acetate
　　g. hydrochloride
gonadotropin, chorionic
Gonic
GonioGel
Goniosol

Gordochom
Gordogesic
Gordomatic
Gordophene
Gormel
Gotamine
gramicidin
Gramimune
Granulex
Gravigen
Grifulvin V
Grillodyne
Grisactin
griseofulvin
Gris-PEG
G-Tussin
G-Tussin DM
Guaiacohist
Guaiacol
Guaiadol
Guaiagesic
Guaiahist
Guaiajen
Guaiamen
guaiapate
Guaifed
guaifenesin
Guaiodol
Guaiphenyl
Guaiphotol
guaithylline

• guamecycline
guanabenz acetate
guanacline sulfate
guanadrel sulfate
guancydine
Guaneran
guanethidine monosulfate
    g. sulfate
guanfacine hydrochloride
guanisoquin sulfate
guanoclor sulfate
guanoctine hydrochloride
guanoxabenz
guanoxan sulfate
guanoxyfen sulfate
Guiamid A.C.
Guiamid D.M.
Guiaphed Elixir
Guistrey Fortis
Gustalac
Gustase
Gustase Plus
gutta percha
Gyn
Gynecort
Gyne-Lotrimin
Gynergen
Gynogen
Gynogen L.A. 10
Gynol 11

H

•hachimycin
halazepam
halazone
Hal-Chlor
Halciderm
halcinonide
Halcion
Haldol
Haldrone
Halenol
Halercol
•halethazole
Haley's M-O
Halodrin
halofantrine hydrochloride
halofenate
halofuginone hydrobromide
Halog
halopemide
haloperidol
    h. decanoate
halopredone acetate
haloprogesterone
haloprogin
•halopyramine
Halorton
Halotestin
Halotex
halothane
Halotussin
Halotussin-DM
•haloxon
halquinols

hamycin
Haniform
Haniplex
Haponal
Harmonyl
Harvaden
Harvatrate A
Harvatropin
Haugase
Hazogel
HBD-UV Test
H-BIG
HC-Derma-Pax
HC-Form
HCG Test
HC-Jel
H-Cort
H.E.A.
Headway
Healon
Heatrol
Heb-Cort
Heb-Cort V
Heb Cream Base
hedaquinium chloride
Hedulin
Heet
hefilcon A
hefilcon B
Heliophan
helium
Hemabex
Hema-Combistix

Hemafate T.D.
Hemaferrin
Hemafolate
Hema-Forte
Hemalive
Hemaspan
Hemaspan-FA
Hemastix
Hemat
Hematest
Hematinic
Hematovals
Hemet
Hemex
hemin
Hemocaine
Hemocyte
Hemocyte-F
Hemocyte Plus
Hemofil
Hemoform
Hemogest
Hemo-Pak
Hemo-Vite
Hemoxygen
Hemozyme
Hemusol HC
heparin sodium
HepatAmine
Hepatolite
Hepato-Scan
Hep-B-Gammagee
Hepfomin
Hep-Forte
Hepicebrin
Hepp-Iron
Hep-Lock
•heptabarbitone

•heptaminol
Heptavax-B
Hepto
Heptuna Plus
Herpecin-L
Herplex
Herplex Liquifilm
Hes-Bic
Hespan
Hesper
Hesper Bitabs
hetacillin
    h. potassium
hetaflur
hetastarch
heteronium bromide
Hetrazan
Hexabax
Hexa-Betalin
hexachlorophene
Hexacrest
Hexaderm
Hexaderm I.Q.
Hexadrol
hexafluorenium bromide
Hexalol
•hexamethonium bromide
Hexamin
•hexamine hippurate
•hexaprofen
•hexapropymate
Hexarutan
Hexasept
Hexate
hexavitamin
hexedine
hexobarbital
hexobendine

Hexopal
•hexoprenaline
hexylcaine hydrochloride
hexylresorcinol
Hexyphen-2
Hexyphen-5
H.H.R.
Hi-Bee
Hibiclens
Hibistat
Hibitane
Hibol
Hi B & C
Hi B Plex
Hi-B Plus
HI-COR 1.0
HI-COR 2.5
Hill Cortac
Hill-Shade
Hipirin
Hi-Po-Vites
Hippuran I 131
Hipputope
Hiprex
Hi-Pro
Hiscatab
Hispril
Hist-A-Balm
Histabid
Hista-C
Histacaps
Histachlor
Hista-Compound No.5
Hista-Derfule
Histadyl
Histadyl E.C.
Histagesic
Histaject

Histalet
Histalet DM
Histalet Forte
Histalet X
Histalog
histamine phosphate
Histan
Hista-Phen
Histarall
Histaspan
Histaspan-D
Histaspan-Plus
Histatab Plus
Histatapp Elixir
Histatapp T.D.
Hista-Vadrin
Hista-Vadrin T.D.
Histerone 100
Histex
histidine
Histolyn-CYL
histoplasmin
Historal
Histor-D
Histor-D Timecelles
Histosal
Histostat-50
Histrey
Histunex
Hi-Temp
Hiwolfia
HMB Gel
HMS Liquifilm
Hold
Homapin
homatropine hydrobromide
    h. methylbromide
Homicebrin

Homogene-S
homosalate
Homo-Tet
•homprenorphine
hoquizil hydrochloride
Hormogen-A
Hormogen Depot
Hournaze
H.P. Acthar Gel
HP Test
HQC
Humafac
Humatin
HuMist
Humorsol
Humulin N
Humulin R
Hurricaine
Hu-Tet
Hyalex
hyaluronidase
Hyamine 1622
Hyamine 3500
Hybec Forte
Hybephen
Hybolin
Hycal
hycanthone
Hycodan
Hycodaphen
Hycoff
Hycoff-A
Hycoff-X
Hycomine
Hycorace
HyCort
Hycotuss
Hydeltra

Hydeltrasol
Hydeltra-T.B.A.
Hydergine
Hydextran
Hydoxin
Hydral
hydralazine hydrochloride
Hydrap-ES
Hydraserp
Hydra-Spray L.A.
Hydrate
Hydrazol
Hydrea
Hydrelt
Hydrex
Hydril
Hydrisalic
Hydrisea Lotion
Hydrisinol
Hydrobexan
Hydro-Chlor
hydrochloric acid
hydrochlorothiazide
Hydro-Cobex
hydrocodone bitartrate
Hydrocil
Hydrocort
hydrocortisone
    h. acetate
    h. butyrate
    h. cypionate
    h. hemisuccinate
    h. sodium phosphate
    h. sodium succinate
    h. valerate
Hydrocortone
Hydrocurve II
HydroDIURIL

hydrofilcon A
hydroflumethiazide
Hydrofol Acid 1655
hydrogen peroxide
Hydrolose
Hydromal
Hydro-Marc
Hydromax
•hydromorphinol
hydromorphone
    hydrochloride
Hydromox
Hydromox R
Hydronol
Hydropane
Hydropel
Hydrophed
Hydrophen
Hydropine #1
Hydropine #2
Hydropres
Hydroquin
hydroquinone
Hydro-Reserp
Hydro-Serp
Hydroserpine
Hydrosol
Hydrosone
•hydrotalcite
Hydro-tex
•hydroxamethocaine
Hydroxo-12
hydroxocobalamin
hydroxyamphetamine
    hydrobromide
hydroxychloroquine
    sulfate
hydroxyphenamate

•hydroxyprocaine
hydroxyprogesterone
    caproate
hydroxypropyl
    methylcellulose
        h. methylcellulose 1828
        h. methylcellulose 2208
        h. methylcellulose 2906
        h. methylcellulose 2910
hydroxystilbamidine
    isethionate
hydroxyurea
hydroxyzine hydrochloride
        h. pamoate
Hydro-Z-50
hy-Flow
Hygroton
Hylate
Hyliver Plus
Hylorel
Hylutin
hymecromone
hymenoptera venom
    extract
•hyoscine methobromide
hyoscyamine
Hyosophen
Hy-Pam
Hypaque
Hypaque-Cysto
Hypaque-DIU
Hypaque-M
Hypaque Meglumine
Hyperab
Hyperetic
HyperHep
Hyperopto
Hypersal

Hyperstat I.V.
Hyperten
Hypertensin
Hyper-Tet
Hypertussis
Hyper-Zem
Hypomins
Hypotears
HypRho-D
Hyprogest 250
•hypromellose
Hyproval P.A.

Hyrexin-50
Hyroxon
Hyserp
Hyskon
Hysone
Hytakerol
Hytinic
Hytinic-UD
Hytone
Hytuss
Hyva
Hyzine-50

I

Iberet
Iberet-500
Iberol
Iberol-F
Ibex
ibopamine
Ibrin
ibufenac
ibuprofen
    i. aluminum
ichthammol
Ichthymall
Ichthyol
ictasol
Ictotest
Icy Hot Balm
I.D. 50
Idarac
Ido-Cortistan
Idotein
idoxuridine

ifosfamide
Igepal CA-630
Igepal CO-430
Igepal CO-630
Igepal CO-730
Igepal CO-880
Iletin
Ilopan
Ilosone
Ilotycin
Ilozyme
I.L.X. Elixir
imafen hydrochloride
Imavate
imcarbofos
Imenol
Imferon
imidecyl iodine
imidocarb hydrochloride
imidoline hydrochloride
imipemide

imipramine hydrochloride
Immuglobin
Immunorex
Imodium
Imogam
•imolamine
Imovax
Impact
Impromen
impromidine hydrochloride
ImunOak
Imuran
Inapsine
Incorpohist
Incremin
indacrinone
indapamide
indeloxazine hydrochloride
Inderal
Inderal LA
Inderide
indigotindisulfonate sodium
indium chlorides In 113m
Indocin
indocyanine green
indomethacin
indoprofen
indoramin
indorenate hydrochloride
indoxole
indriline hydrochloride
Infacaps A & D
Infalyte
Infantol Pink
Infantovit
Infatuss
Infatussis
Infiltrase

Inflamase
Inflamase Forte
infraRUB
INH
Inhiston
Inkalyte
Innovar
Inocor
•inosine pranobex
inositol niacinate
Inpersol
•inproquone
Inserfem
Insta-Glucose
Inst-E-Vite
Insulatard NPH
insulin
    dalanated i.
    globin zinc i.
    human i.
    Humulin N
    Humulin R
    I 125 i.
    I 131 i.
    Iletin I
    isophane i.
    Lentard i.
    Lente Iletin I
    Monotard i.
    neutral i.
    protamine zinc i.
    Semilente Iletin I
    Semitard i.
    Ultralente i.
    Ultratard i.
    zinc i.
Intal
Intensin

Intercept
interferon
Intralipid
Intra-Sul
intrazole
intriptyline hydrochloride
Intron-C
Intropin
inulin
Inversine
iobenzamic acid
iocarmate meglumine
iocarmic acid
iocetamic acid
Iocon
Iocortar
iodamide
    i. meglumine
Iodex
iodine
iodipamide
    i. meglumine
    i. sodium I 131
iodoantipyrine I 131
iodocetylic acid I 123
iodochlorhydroxyquin
iodocholesterol I 131
Iodocort
iodohippurate sodium I 123
    i. sodium I 125
    i. sodium I 131
Iodo-Niacin
Iodopen
iodopyracet I 125
iodopyracet I 131
iodoquinol
Iodosone
Iodotope I 131

Iodotope Therapeutic
iodoxamate meglumine
iodoxamic acid
ioglicic acid
ioglucol
ioglucomide
ioglycamic acid
iogulamide
iohexol
iomethin I 125
iomethin I 131
Ionamin
Ionax
Ionil
Ionosol D-CM
iopamidol
iopanoic acid
Iophed
iophendylate
Ioprep
ioprocemic acid
iopronic acid
iopydol
iopydone
iosefamic acid
ioseric acid
iosulamide meglumine
iosumetic acid
iotasul
iotetric acid
iothalamate meglumine
    i. sodium I 125
    i. sodium I 131
    i. sodium
iothalamic acid
iotroxic acid
iotyrosine I 131
ioxaglate meglumine

ioxaglate (*continued*)
    i. sodium
ioxaglic acid
ioxotrizoic acid
ipecac
ipexidine mesylate
ipodate calcium
    i. sodium
ipratropium bromide
iprindole
•iproniazid
ipronidazole
Ipropran
iproxamine hydrochloride
•ipsalazide
Ipsatol
Ipsatol-DM
Ircon
Ircon-FA
iridium Ir 192
Irigate
Irodex
Irolong II
Iromide
Iromin-G
Ironate-B
iron dextran
    i. sorbitex
isamoxole
Ismelin
Ismotic
Isobarb
Iso-Bid
isobucaine hydrochloride
Isobutal
isobutamben
Isocal

Isocal HCN
isocarboxazid
Isoclor
isoconazole
Isocrin
Isodettes
Isodine
isoetharine
    i. hydrochloride
    i. mesylate
Isofedrol
Isofil
isoflupredone acetate
isoflurane
isoflurophate
Isogard
Isogen
Isoject
Isolate
isoleucine
isomerol
Isomil
Isomil SF
Isomil SF 20
isomylamine hydrochloride
isoniazid
Isopacin
Isopaque 440
Iso-Par
Iso-Perazine
isophane
Isophed
•isoprednidene
•isoprenaline
isopropamide iodide
isopropyl alcohol
    i. myristate
    i. palmitate

Isopro T.D.
isoproterenol hydrochloride
   i. sulfate
Isoptin
Isopto Alkaline
Isopto Atropine
Isopto Carbachol
Isopto Carpine
Isopto Cetamide
Isopto Cetapred
Isopto Eserine
Isopto Frin
Isopto Homatropine
Isopto Hyoscine
Isopto P-ES
Isopto Plain
Isopto Tears
Isordil

Isordil Tembids
isosorbide
isosorbide dinitrate
•isosorbide mononitrate
isostearyl alcohol
isosulfan blue
Isotein HN
isotretinoin
Isovex-100
Isovue
isoxepac
isoxicam
isoxsuprine hydrochloride
Isuprel
Ivadantin
ivermectin
Ivy-Chex
Ivy-Rid

J

Janimine
Janupap
Jayron
Jecto Sal
Jel Drox
Jenamicin
Jen-Balm
Jen-Diril
Jenkaps
Jen-Lax

Jensenex
Jen-Vite
Jeri-Lotion
Jiffy
J-Liberty
Johnson's Medicated Powder
josamycin
Junicoid
juniper tar
Junyer-All

K

Kabikinase
kalafungin
Kalcinate
•kallidinogenase
Kalol
Kamabel
Kamagel
Kamfolene
Kamoran
Kanalka
kanamycin sulfate
Kank-a
Kankex
Kanpectin-P
Kantrex
Kanulase
Kaocasil
Kaochlor
Kaochlor-Eff
Kaochlor S-F
Kaodene
Kaodonna PG
kaolin
Kaon
Kaon-Cl
Kaon-Cl-10
Kaon-Cl 20%
Kao-Nor
Kaopectate
Kao-Pectin
Kapectolin
Ka-Pek
Kapinal

Kappadione
Karidium
Karigel
Kari-Rinse
kasal
Kasof
Ka-Thal-Pec
Kato
Kavacaps
Kavrin
Kaybovite 1000
Kay-B-Plex
Kay Ciel
Kayexalate
Kaypectol
Kaytrate
Kaytron
KBP/O
K-C
Kedrin
Keelamin
Keff
Keflex
Keflin
Kefzol
Kelatrate
Kemadrin
Kenac
Kenacort
Kenahist-S.A.
Kenalog
Kenalog-H
Kenalone

Kenpectin
Ken-Tuss
Keotin
Keralyt
Keri
Kerid Ear Drops
Kerodex
Kessadrox
Kesso-Bamate
Kessodanten
Kessodrate
Kesso-Mycin
Kesso-Pen
Kessotapp
Kesso-Tetra
Kestrin
Kestrone
Ketaject
Ketalar
ketamine hydrochloride
ketanserin
Ketaset
ketazocine
ketazolam
kethoxal
ketipramine fumarate
•ketobemidone
Ketochol
ketoconazole
Keto-Diastix
Ketolan
ketoprofen
ketorfanol
ketotifen fumarate
Ketostix
Key-Plex
Key-Pred-25
Key-Pred Plus

Key-Pred SP
K-Feron
K-Flex
K-Forte
K-G Elixir
Kiddisan
KIE Syrup
Kinder-Dare
Kinesed
Kinevac
kitasamycin
Klaron
Klavikordal
Klebcil
Kleer Loz
K-Lor
Klor-10%
Klor-Con
Klor-Con/25
Kloromin
Klorvess
Klotrix
K-Lyte
K-Lyte/Cl
K-Lyte/Cl-50
Koate
Kodet SE
Kolantyl
Kolephrin DM
Kolephrin NN
Kolyum
Komed
Komed HC
Konakion
Kondremul
Konlax
Konsto
Konsyl

Konyne
Kophane
Korigesic
Korizol
Koromex
Koromex II
Koromex II-A
Korostatin
Koro-Sulf
Kort
Korum
K-P
K-Pek

K-Phen
K-Phos Neutral
Kronofed-A Jr. Kronocaps
Kronofed-A Kronocaps
Kronohist
krypton clathrate Kr 85
krypton Kr 81m
K-Tab
Kudrox
Kutapressin
Kutrase
Ku-Zyme HP
Kwell

L

LA-12
labetalol hydrochloride
LaBID
Labstix
Lacotein
Lacril
Lacri-Lube S.O.P.
Lacrisert
LactAid
lactic acid
LactiCare
Lactinex
Lactocal-F
lactose
lactulose
L.A. Dezone
L.A.E. 20
L.A. Formula
Laktomol
Lamine

Lamotane-X
Lanabac
Lanabarb
Lanabee-C
Lanabrom Elixir
Lanaburn
Lanacane
Lanacillin
Lanacort
Lanamins
Lanaphilic
Lanased
•lanatoside C
Lanatrate
Lanatuss
Lanaurine
Lanavite
Lanazets
Lan-E
Lanestrin

Laniazid
Lannates Elixir
Lanokalin
lanolin
Lanoline
Lanolor
Lanophyllin
Lanophyllin-GG
Lanoplex Elixir
Lanorinal
Lanoxin
Lanteen Jelly
Lantrisul
Lanvisone
Lapav
Lapav Graduals
lapyrium chloride
Lardet
Largon
Larobec
Larodopa
Larotid
Larylgan
Larynex
lasalocid
Lasan
Lasix
Lassar's paste
•latamoxef disodium
Laudacin
•laudexium methylsulphate
laureth 4
laureth 9
laureth 105
Lauro
•laurolinium acetate
lauryl isoquinolinium
   bromide

Lavacol
Lavatar
Lavema
Lavogent
Lavoptik
Lavoris
Laxatab
Laxatyl
Laxinate 100
Laxogen
LC-65
L-Caine
L-Caine E
L.C.D.
L-Cysteine HCl
Lec-E-Plex
lecithin
Lec-Kelp
Leder-BP Sequels
Ledercillin VK
Leder-CPI Sequels
Lederplex
Lemiserp
Lemivite-M FCT
Lenate
leniquinsin
lenperone
Lensen
Lensine
Lens-Mate
Lensrins
Lens-Wet
Lentard
Lente
Lente Iletin
Lente Iletin I
Lente Iletin II
lergotrile

lergotrile (*continued*)
   l. mesylate
Lerton Ovules
Les-Cav
Lesterol
Le-Test
Lethopherol
letimide hydrochloride
leucine
leucovorin calcium
Leukeran
leukocyte typing serum
leuprolide acetate
levallorphan tartrate
levamfetamine succinate
Levamine
levamisole hydrochloride
•levamphetamine succinate
Leviron
levobunolol hydrochloride
levodopa
Levo-Dromoran
levofuraltadone
Levoid
levomethadyl acetate
•levomethorphan
•levomoramide
levonantradol hydrochloride
levonordefrin
levonorgestrel
Levopa
Levophed
Levoprome
levopropoxyphene napsylate
levopropylcillin potassium
levorphanol tartrate
Levothroid
levothyroxine sodium

levoxadrol hydrochloride
Levsin
Levsinex
Levucal
Lexavite
Lexocort
Lexor
Lextron
Lextron Ferrous Pulvules
Lextron F.G. Pulvules
L.F.B. 12-100
L-Glutavite
Libidinal
Libigen
Librax
Libritabs
Librium
Licoplex
Licoplex DS
licryfilcon A
licryfilcon B
Licryl-55
Licryl-70
Lidaform-HC
Lida-Mantle
lidamidine hydrochloride
Lidanar
Lidex
Lidex-E
lidocaine
   l. hydrochloride
lidofenin
lidofilcon A
lidofilcon B
lidoflazine
Lidoject-1
Lidoject-2
LidoPen

Lidosporin Otic
Lidoxide
Life Plex
Lifer-B
lifibrate
Lifocort-100
Lifoject
Lifol-B
Lifolbex
Lifolex
Lifomin
•lignocaine
Limbitrol
Limbo
lime
Limit
Lincocin
lincomycin
    l. hydrochloride
lindane
linogliride fumarate
Lioresal
liothyronine I 125
liothyronine I 131
liothyronine sodium
liotrix
Lipiodol
Lipivas
Lipkote
Lipo-Art
Lipo-B-C
Lipoflavonoid
Lipo Gantrisin
Lipogen
Lipo-Hepin
Lipo-K
Lipoleit
Lipo-Lutin

Lipomul IV
Lipo-Nicin
Liponol
Liposyn
Lipotin
Lipotriad
Lipovite
Liquaemin
Liquamar
Liquapen
Liqui-Doss
Liquid Pred
Liquifilm Forte
Liquifilm Tears
Liquimat
Liqui-Nox
Liquiprin
Liquitussin
Liquitussin A-C
Liquophylline
Lisacort
Listerex
Listerine
Lithane
lithium carbonate
    l. citrate
    l. hydroxide
Lithobid
Lithonate
Lithostat
Lithotabs
Liva
Livec
Liver
Liverbex
Livergran
Liv-Fer-B
Liv-Fer-Blex

Livifol
Livi-Plex
Livitamin
Livitol
Livonamine
Livorex
Livroben
Livtrinsic
Lixaminol
Lixaminol AT
Lixoil
Lixolin
L-Lysine
Lobana
Lobana Peri-Gard
lobendazole
Lobidram
Locane
Locoid
Locorten
Locron P
Lodosyn
lodoxamide ethyl
    l. tromethamine
Lodrane
Loestrin 21
Loestrin Fe
Lofenalac
•lofendazam
Lofene
lofentanil oxalate
•lofepramine
lometraline hydrochloride
lomofungin
Lomotil
lomustine
Lonalac
Loniten

Lo/Ovral
loperamide hydrochloride
Lopid
•loprazolam
Lopressor
Loprox
Lopurin
Loqua
lorajmine hydrochloride
lorazepam
lorbamate
lorcainide hydrochloride
Lorelco
Lorfan
lormetazepam
Lorothidol
Loroxide
Loroxide-HC
Lorphen
lorzafone
Lo-Sal
Lo Tense
Lotio-P
Lotrimin
Lo-Trol
Lo-Trop
Lotusate
Lotussin
Lowila
Low-Quel
loxapine
    l. succinate
Loxitane
Loxon
•loxtidine
Lozol
Lubinol
Lubriderm

lucanthone hydrochloride
Lucidon
Ludiomil
Luf-Iso
Lufyllin
Lufyllin-EPG
Lufyllin-GG
Lugol's solution
Luminal
Luride
Luride Lozi-Tabs
Lustozyme
Lutocylol
Lutolin-F
Lutolin-S
lyapolate sodium
lycetamine
Lycolan
lydimycin
•lymecycline

lymphogranuloma venereum
    antigen
LymphoScan
lynestrenol
Lynoral
Lyophrin
Lyopine
Lyovac
Lypo-B
lypressin
•lysergide
lysine
    l. acetate
    l. hydrochloride
Lysmins
Lysodren
lysostaphin
•lysuride
Lyteers
Lytren

M

Maalox
Maalox Plus
Maalox TC
Macrodantin
Macrodex
•Macrogol 400
•Macrogol 4000
Macrospherical 95
Madopa
mafenide
    m. acetate
mafilcon A

magaldrate
Magan
Magdrox
Maglagel
Mag-5
Magma Alba
Magmalin
Magnacal
Magnacort
Magnagel
Magnalets
Magnalum

Magnamycin
Magnased
Magnatril
magnesium
magnesium aluminum silicate
 m. carbonate
 m. chloride
 m. citrate
 m. gluconate
 m. hydroxide
 m. oxide
 m. phosphate
 m. salicylate
 m. sulfate
 m. trisilicate
Magnex
Magnipin
Magoleum
Magonate
Magora
Mag-Ox
Magsal
Malatal
malathion
malethamer
Maliasin
Mallamint
Mallergan
Mallergan-VC
Mallisol
Mallo-Pectin
Mallopress
Malogel
Malogen CYP 200
Malogen L.A. 200
Malotuss
Maltsupex
Mammol

Manalax
Mandelamine
Mandex
Mandol
manganese chloride
 m. sulfate
Mangatrace
mannitol
 m. hexanitrate
•mannomustine
Manola
Manotensin
Mansil
Mantadil
Mantomide
Manvitol
Manzan
Maolate
Maox
maprotiline
Maracid-2
Maranox
Marax
Marax DF
Marazide
Marazide II
Marbec
Marblen
Marcaine
Mardon
MarEPA
Maretin
Marezine
Marflex
Margesic Compound 65
Marhist
Marmine
Marnal

Marplan
Mar-Tonic
Masse
Massengill
Masterone
Materna 1.60
Maternavite
Matromycin
Matulane
Maxafil
Maxamag
Maxibolin
Maxicam
Maxidex
Maxiflor
Maxigesic
Maxipen
Maxitate
Maxitrol
Maygel
maytansine
Mazanor
mazindol
Mazon
MBF
M-Caps
M-Cillin
MCT
MD-76
Measurin
Mebaral
mebendazole
mebeverine hydrochloride
•mebezonium iodide
•mebhydrolin
mebrofenin
Mebroin
Mebryl

mebutamate
Mecadox
mecamylamine hydrochloride
mechlorethamine
    hydrochloride
Mechol
Mecholyl
Meclan
meclizine hydrochloride
meclocycline
    m. sulfosalicylate
meclofenamate sodium
meclofenamic acid
•meclofenoxate
Meclomen
mecloqualone
meclorisone dibutyrate
•meclozine
mecobalamin
mecrylate
Medache
Meda-Hist
Medalox
Med-Apap
Meda-Tex
Meda-Tuss
medazepam hydrochloride
Med-Depo
Mediatric
Medibrin-T
Medicaine
Medi-Cil
Medi-Con
Mediconet
Medigesic
Medihaler-Duo
Medihaler-Epi
Medihaler-Ergotamine

Medihaler-Iso
Medipak
Mediplast
Mediplex Tabules
Medique
Medi-Quik
Medi-Spas
Medi-Tal
Medi-Tec 90
Meditussin-X
Medizinc
Medotar
Medralone-40
Medralone-80
medrogestone
Medrol
Medrol ADT Pak
Medrol Dosepak
Medrol Enpak
medronate disodium
medronic acid
Medrone
medroxalol
   m. hydrochloride
medroxyprogesterone
  acetate
medrysone
Med-Tane
Med-Tapp
mefenamic acid
mefenidil
   m. fumarate
mefenorex hydrochloride
mefexamide
mefloquine
Mefoxin
mefruside
Mega-B

Megace
Megadose
megalomicin potassium
  phosphate
Mega-Vita
megestrol acetate
meglumine
meglutol
•meladrazine
Melanate
•melarsonyl potassium
•melarsoprol
Melasol
melengestrol acetate
Melfiat
Melfiat-105 Unicelles
melitracen hydrochloride
melizame
Mellaril
melphalan
memotine hydrochloride
menabitan hydrochloride
menadiol sodium
  diphosphate
menadione
   m. sodium bisulfite
•menbutone
Menest
Menic
Meni-D
Meningovax-AC
menoctone
Menoject-LA
Menolyn
Menomune-A,C,Y,W
menotropins
Menrium 5-2
Menrium 5-4

Menrium 10-4
Menstress
Menta-Bal
Mentalert
Menthalgesic
menthol
Mentholatum
Mentholin
Mentrolz
meobentine sulfate
Meonine
mepartricin
mepenzolate bromide
Mepergan
meperidine hydrochloride
mephentermine sulfate
mephenytoin
mephobarbital
Mephyton
Mepiben
•mepiprazole
mepivacaine hydrochloride
Mepred
meprednisone
Mepriam
meprobamate
Mepro Compound
Meprocon
Meprogesic
Meprospan
Meprotabs
•meprothixol
meprylcaine hydrochloride
•meptazinol
•mepyramine
mequidox
Mequin
mercaptomerin sodium

mercaptopurine
Mercodol
Mercresin
mercufenol chloride
Mercurochrome
Mercurol
mercury, ammoniated
Mercutheolin
Mercuzanthin
merisoprol acetate Hg 197
merisoprol acetate Hg 203
merisoprol Hg 197
Merital
Meritene
Merlenate
Merodicein
Merphenyl
Mersa
Mersene
Mersol
Merthiolate
Meruvax II
Mervaldin
Mervan
Mesantoin
meseclazone
mesifilcon A
Meso Lens
Mesopin
mesoridazine
    m. besylate
mesterolone
Mestinon
mestranol
mesuprine hydrochloride
metabromsalan
•metacetamol
Metahydrin

metalol hydrochloride
Metalone T.B.A.
Metamine
Metamucil
Metandren
Metandren Linguets
Metaphedrin
Metaprel
metaproterenol sulfate
metaraminol
Metasep
Metatensin
•metazocine
Metazol
Meted
meteneprost
metformin
Meth
methacholine chloride
methacycline
     m. hydrochloride
methadone hydrochloride
Methadose
methadyl acetate
Methagual
Methakote
Methalate
Methalgen
methallibure
methalthiazide
Methampex
•methamphazone
•methandienone
methandrostenolone
methantheline bromide
methapyrilene fumarate
     m. hydrochloride
methaqualone

methaqualone (*continued*)
     m. hydrochloride
metharbital
•metharbitone
Methazine
methazolamide
Meth-Choline
methdilazine
     m. hydrochloride
methenamine
     m. hippurate
     m. mandelate
methenolone acetate
     m. enanthate
Methergine
methetoin
methicillin sodium
methimazole
methiodal sodium
methionine
Methioplex
methisazone
Methischol
Methium
methixene hydrochloride
Methnite
methocarbamol
Methocel A,E,F,K
methohexital
     m. sodium
•methoin
methopholine
Methopto Forte
Methosarb
methotrexate
     m. sodium
methotrimeprazine
methoxamine hydrochloride

methoxsalen
methoxyflurane
methoxyphenamine
  hydrochloride
Methral
methscopolamine bromide
methsuximide
Methulose
methyclothiazide
Methydiol
methyl
  m. alcohol
  m. amylketone
  m. anthranilate
  m. benzene
  m. chloride
  m. cyanide
  m. ethyl-maleicimid
  m. ethyl-pyrrole
  m. eugenol
  m. heptenone
  m. hydride
  m. hydroxy-furfurol
  m. iodide
  m. isobutyl ketone
  m. methacrylate
  m. palmoxirate
  m. salicylate
  m. sulfonate
  m. telluride
methylatropine nitrate
methylbenzethonium chloride
methylcellulose
•methylchromone
•methyldesorphine
methyldopa
methyldopate hydrochloride
methylene blue

methylergonovine maleate
Methylgesic
methylphenidate
  hydrochloride
methylprednisolone
  m. acetate
  m. hemisuccinate
  m. sodium phosphate
  m. sodium succinate
methyltestosterone
methylthiouracil
methynodiol diacetate
methyprylon
•methyridene
methysergide
  m. maleate
metiamide
metiapine
Meticortelone
Meticorten
Meti-Derm
Metimyd
metioprim
metizoline hydrochloride
metkephamid acetate
metoclopramide
  hydrochloride
metocurine iodide
metogest
metolazone
metopimazine
Metopirone
metoprine
metoprolol
  m. tartrate
metoquizine
metoserpate hydrochloride
Metra

Metrazol
Metreton
•metriphonate
metrizamide
metrizoate sodium
Metrogesic
Metro IV
Metrojen
metronidazole
    m. hydrochloride
    m. phosphate
Metryl
Metubine
meturedepa
Metycaine
metyrapone
    m. tartrate
metyrosine
Mevanin-C
Mevatinic-C
Mexate
•mexenone
Mexitil
mexrenoate potassium
Mexsana
Mezlin
mezlocillin
Mg-PLUS
mianserin hydrochloride
mibolerone
Mi-Bon
Mi-Bon-T
Mi-Cebrin
Micofur
miconazole nitrate
Micoren
MICRhoGAM
Micrainin

Micrin
Microcort
Micro Dry
Micro-K
Microlipid
Micronase
microNefrin
Micronor
Microsol
Microstix-Nitrite
Microstix-3
Microsul
Microsul-A
Microsulfon
Microsyn
MicroTrak
midaflur
Midahist DH
Midamor
Midaneed
Midatane
Midatane DC
Midatap
midazolam hydrochloride
    m. maleate
midodrine hydrochloride
Midol
Miflex
Migergot P-B
Migrade
Migral
•mikamycin
Milco-Zyme
milenperone
milipertine
Milkinol
Milontin
Milontin Kapseals

Milpath
Milprem
Miltown
Miltrate
mimbane hydrochloride
minaxolone
•minepentate
mineral oil
Min-Hema
Mini-Lix
Minipress
Minitec
Minizide
Minocin
minocycline
    m. hydrochloride
Minocyn
minoxidil
Minro-Plex
Mintezol
Mint-O-Mag
Minut-Rub
Min-Viteral
Miocel
Miochol
Miostat
Miradon
Miral
MiraSol
mirincamycin hydrochloride
misonidazole
misoprostol
Mission Prenatal F.A.
Mission Prenatal H.P.
Mitaban
Mi-Theric
Mithracin
mithramycin

mitindomide
•mitobronitol
mitocarcin
•mitoclomine
mitocromin
mitogillin
mitomalcin
mitomycin
•mitopodozide
mitosper
mitotane
Mitrolan
Mity-Mycin
Mity-Quin
Mivert
mixidine
Mixtard
Mizyme
M-M-R II
Mn-PLUS
Moban
Mobidin
Mobigesic
Mobisyl
modaline sulfate
Modane
Modane Soft
Moderil
Modicon
Modrenal
Moducal
Moduretic
Moebiquin
Mogadon
M.O., Haley's
Molatoc
Molatoc-CST
molinazone

molindone hydrochloride
Mol-Iron
Mollifene
molsidomine
Molypen
Momentum
Monacrin
monensin
Monistat
Monistat-Derm
Monistat 7
Monobase
monobenzone
Monocete
Monochlor
Monocortin
Monodral
Mono-Gesic
Monojel
Monopar
•monosulfiram
Monotard
Mono-Vacc
Monteban
morantel tartrate
•morazone
Morco
moricizine
morniflumate
Moroline
morphine sulfate
morrhuate sodium
Mor-Tussin P.E.
Motion-Aid
Motofen
motretinide
Motrin
Movicol

moxalactam disodium
Moxam
•moxaverine
moxazocine
•moxipraquine
moxnidazole
Moyco
M-Prednisol-40
M-2 Protocol
M/Rinse
M-R-Vax II
MSG-600
M.T.E.-5
Mucillium
Mucilose
Mucogel
Mucomyst
Mucomyst-10
Mudd
Mudrane
Mudrane-2
Mudrane GG
Mudrane GG-2
Multa-Gen 12
Multicebrin
Multifluor
Multi-Germ
Multigest
Multilex-T/M
Multi-Scrub
Multitest CMI
Multi-Vites
Multorex
Mulvidren-F
Mumpsvax
Murcil
Muriamic
Murine

Murine Plus
Muripsin
Murocel
Murocoll-2
Muro 128
Muro's Opcon-A
Muro Tears
Mustargen
Musterole
•mustine
Mutamycin
muzolimine
M.V.C. 9 + 3
MVC Plus
M.V.I.-12
Myadec
Myambutol
Mycelex
Mycelex-G
Mychel
Mycifradin
Myciguent
Myci-Spray
Mycitracin
Mycolog
mycophenolic acid
My Cort
Mycostatin
Myco Triacet
Mydfrin
Mydrapred

Mydriacyl
Mygel
Myidone
Mylanta
Mylanta-II
Mylaxen
Myleran
Mylicon
Mylicon-80
Mylosar
Myobid
Myocalm
Myochrysine
Myoflex
Myoforte
Myolin
Myophen
Myordil
Myosal
Myprozine
•myralact
Myringacaine
•myrophine
Mysoline
Mysteclin-F
Mysuran
Mytelase
Mytrate
Mytrex
Myverol
M-Z

N

nabazenil
nabilone
nabitan hydrochloride
naboctate hydrochloride
•nabumetone
Nacrem
nadide
nadolol
•nafazatrom
Nafcil
nafcillin sodium
nafenopin
nafomine malate
nafoxidine hydrochloride
nafronyl oxalate
naftalofos
•naftazone
•naftidrofuryl
naftifine hydrochloride
Nagest
Nalate
nalbuphine hydrochloride
Naldecon
Naldecon-CX
Naldecon-DX
Naldecon-EX
Naldegesic
Naldelate
Naldetuss
Nalfon
nalidixate sodium
nalidixic acid
Nalline

Nallpen
nalmefene
nalmexone hydrochloride
nalorphine hydrochloride
naloxone hydrochloride
naltrexone
namoxyrate
Nandrobolic
Nandrobolic L.A.
Nandrolin
nandrolone cyclotate
    n. decanoate
    n. phenpropionate
nantradol hydrochloride
Naotin
naphazoline hydrochloride
Naphcon-A
Naphcon Forte
Naplopan
Napril Plateau
Naprosyn
naproxen
    n. sodium
naproxol
Naptrate
Naqua
Naquival
naranol hydrochloride
narasin
Narcan
Nardil
Narspan
Nasahist

Nasalcrom
Nasalide
Nasdro
Nasophen
Natabec-FA Kapseals
Natabec Rx Kapseals
Natacomp-FA
Natacyn
Natafort Filmseal
Natalins Rx
natamycin
Nata-Par
Nataplex-C
Naturacil
Natur-Aid
Naturetin
Naturil
Natur-Lax
Naturvue
Nausetrol
Navane
Navaron
Nazac
N.B.P.
ND Clear T.D.
ND-Gesic
ND-Hist
ND-Stat
•nealbarbitone
Nebcin
nebramycin
Nebs
Nebu-Prel
Nechlorin
Nectavite-M
nefopam hydrochloride
Negatan
NegGram

Nembutal
Neo-Antergan
Neo-Betalin 12
Neobiotic
Neocaine
Neo-Calglucon
Neo-Castaderm
Neocholan
Neo-Cobefrin
Neo-Cort-Dome
Neo-Cortef
Neo-Cultol
Neocurb
Neocurtasal
Neo-Cutone
Neocylate
NeoDecadron
NeoDecaspray
Neo-Delta-Cortef
NeoFed
Neo-Flo
Neo-Gerastan
Neo-Hydeltrasol
Neo-Hydro
Neolax
Neo-Lep 3
Neolin
Neoloid
Neomark
Neo-Medrol
neomycin palmitate
neomycin sulfate
neomycin undecylenate
Neo-Oxylone
Neopham
Neophyl
Neo-Polycin
Neoquess

Neo-Rhiban
Neosar
Neoscan
Neosone
Neosorb
Neosporin
Neosporin-G
Neo-Spray
Neostig
neostigmine bromide
neostigmine methylsulfate
Neo-Synalar
Neo-Synephrine
Neo-Synephrine 12 Hour
Neo-Synephrine II
Neo-Synephrinol
Neotal
Neo-Tears
Neotep Granucaps
Neo-Thrycex
Neothylline
Neothylline-GG
Neotrizine
Neo-Trobex
Neotrol
Neotuss-PT
NeoVadrin B-Complex 50
Neo-Vadrin Centra-Vite
NeoVicaps
Neozin
Nephramine
Nephrox
Neptazane
nequinate
Nervine
Nervocaine
Nesacaine
Nesacaine-CE

Nestabs
Nestabs FA
Nethaphyl
netilmicin sulfate
Netromycin
Neuramate
Neurate-400
Neut
Neutracomp
Neutralox
neutramycin
Neutra-Phos
Neutra-Phos-K
Neutrogena
Nevrotose
Newphrine
nexeridine hydrochloride
NGT
Niac
Niacal
niacin
niacinamide
Nialex
Niamid
Niapent
Niarb
Niatinic
Nibesol
nibroxane
Nicalex
•nicametate
•nicarbazin
nicardipine hydrochloride
nicergoline
•niceritrol
Niclocide
•niclofolan
niclosamide

Nico-400
Nicobid
Nicocap
•nicocodine
•nicodicodine
Nicolar
Nico-Metrazol
nicorandil
Nico-Span
•nicotinamide
Nicotinex
•nicotinic acid
nicotinyl alcohol
•nicoumalone
Nico-Vert
Nicozide
Nicozin-C
Nicozol
nifedipine
•nifenazone
Niferex Forte
Niferex-150
Niferex-PN
nifluridide
nifungin
nifuradene
nifuraldezone
nifuratel
nifuratrone
nifurdazil
nifurimide
nifurmerone
nifurpirinol
nifurquinazol
nifursemizone
nifursol
nifurthiazole
•nifurtimox

Nigrin
Nil
Nilain
Niloden
nimazone
nimidane
nimodipine
•nimorazole
Ninhydrin
Nionate
Niong
Nioric
Nipride
Niratron
niridazole
Niron
Nisaval
nisbuterol mesylate
Niscort
Nisentil
nisobamate
nisoldipine
Nisolone-40
nisoxetine
Ni-Span
nisterime acetate
nitarsone
nithiamide
nitrafudam hydrochloride
nitralamine hydrochloride
nitramisole hydrochloride
nitrazepam
Nitrazine paper
Nitrazone
•nitrefazole
nitrendipine
Nitrex
Nitrin

Nitro-Bid IV
Nitro-Bid 2.5
Nitro-Bid 6.5
Nitro-Bid 9
Nitrocap
Nitrocap T.D.
nitrocycline
nitrodan
Nitrodisc
Nitro-Dur
nitrofurantoin
nitrofurazone
nitroglycerin
Nigroglyn
Nitrol
Nitrolin
nitromersol
nitromide
nitromifene citrate
Nitronal
Nitronet
Nitrong
Nitropress
nitroscanate
Nitrospan
Nitrostat
Nitrostat IV
Nitrostat SR
Nitro T.D.
nitrous oxide
Nitrovas
•nitroxoline
nivazol
Nivea
nivimedone sodium
nizatidine
Nizoral
N-Multistix

N-N
Nobese
nocodazole
Noctec
No Doz
nogalamycin
No Gest
Nokane
Nolahist
Nolamine
nolinium bromide
Noludar
Nolvadex
nomifensine maleate
•nonabine
nonoxynol 4
nonoxynol 9
nonoxynol 15
nonoxynol 30
Nonsul Jelly
noracymethadol
    hydrochloride
Noralac
Norazine
norbolethone
•norbutrine
Norcet
•norcodeine
nordefrin hydrochloride
Nordette
Nordryl
Norel Plus
norepinephrine bitartrate
norethindrone
    n. acetate
•norethisterone
norethynodrel
Norflex

norflurane
Norgesic
Norgesic Forte
norgestimate
norgestomet
norgestrel
Noriday
Norimex-Plus
Norinyl
Norisodrine
Norlac
Norlac RX
Norlestrin 21
Norlestrin Fe
•norlevorphanol
Nor-Lief
Norlutate
Norlutin
Normacid
Normaderm
Normatane
Normatane DC
Nor-Mil
Normosol-M 900 CAL
Normosol-R
Normosol-R/K
Normotensin
Norocaine
Norodin
Norophylline
Noroxine
Norozol
Norpace
Norpanth
Norphyl
•norpipanone
Norpramin
Nor-Pred S

Nor-Pred T.B.A.
Nor-Q.D.
Nor-Tet
nortriptyline hydrochloride
Nortussin
NoSalt
noscapine
Noscaps
nosiheptide
Noskote
Nospaz
Nostril
Nostrilla
Nostyn
Novafed
Novafed A
Novahistine
Novahistine DH
Novahistine DMX
Novahistine Fortis
Novahistine LP
Novahistine Melet
Novaldin
Novamine
Novamor
Novastat-W
Novatuss
Novazole
Novocain
Novocell
Novrad
•noxiptyline
•noxythiolin
Noxzema
NP-27
NPH Iletin
NPH Iletin I
NTZ

Nubain
Nuclomin
Nucofed
Nucorsal
Nu-Dispoz
Nu-Flow
Nu-Iron 150
Nu-Iron-Plus Elixir
Nu-Iron-V
Nujol
Nu'Leven
Nulicaine
Nullapons
Nullo
Nul-Tach
Numal
Numorphan
Numotizine
Numzident
Num-zit
Nupercainal
Nupercaine
N-Uristix
Nurolon
Nursoy
Nu-Thera
Nutracort

Nutraderm
Nutrajel
Nutramag
Nutrament
Nutramigen
Nutramin
Nutraplus
Nutrasweet
Nutricol
Nitricon
Nutri-Drops
Nutrizyme
Nuvac
Nydrazid
Nylamine
nylestriol
nylidrin hydrochloride
Nylmerate II
NyQuil
Nyral
Nysolone
Nystaform
Nystaform-HC
nystatin
Nytilax
Nytol

O

Oasis
Obacin
Obalan
Obepar
Obephen
Obermine

Obestat 75
Obestat 150
Obestin-30
Obetrim
Obetrol
Obetrol-10

Obetrol-20
Obeval
Obezine
obidoxime chloride
Oblate
Obrical
Obrical-F
Obron-6
Obtundia
Ob-Vit
OC-250
Ocean Nasal Mist
Ocean Plus Mist
ocrylate
octabenzone
octamethyl
  pyrophosphoramide
Octarex
•octatropine methylbromide
•octaverine
Octavims
octazamide
octenidine hydrochloride
octicizer
Octin
Octocaine
octocrylene
octodrine
octoxynol 9
octriptyline phosphate
octrizole
ocufilcon A
ocufilcon B
ocufilcon C
Ocusert Pilo-20
Odalate
Odara
Odex

Odin CR
Odor-Scrip
Off-Ezy
Ogen
Oilatum
Oil-O-Sol
olaflur
•olaquindox
Olaxin
oleic acid I 125
oleovitamin A and D
Ominal
Omnibel
Omnibese
Omnicol
Omnigesic
Omnihemin
Omninatal
Omnipen
Omnipen-N
Omnitabs
Omnitrate
Omuretic
Oncovin
One-A-Day
One Solution
Onset-5
Onset-10
Ontosein
Operand
Ophthaine
Ophthalgan
Ophtha P/S
Ophthetic
Ophthochlor
Ophthocort
opipramol hydrochloride
Opticaps

Opti-clean
Optilets-500
Optilets-M-500
Optimine
Optimyd
opipramol hydrochloride
opium
Opt-Ease
Optef
Op-Thal-Zin
Opthocort
Opticaps
Optigene
Optimine
Optimyd
Optised
Optivites
ORA 5
Orabase
Orabilex
Oracin
Oradex-C
Oraflex
Oragrafin
Orahist
Orajel
Oralphyllin
Ora-Lutin
Oraminic
Orapav Timecelles
Oraphen-PD
Orapin
Orasone
Oraspan
Ora-Testryl
Oratrast
Oratrol
Oratuss

Oravue
Orazinc
Orbetic
Orbit
•orciprenaline
orconazole nitrate
Orenzyme
Oretic
Oreticyl
Oreticyl Forte
Oreton
Orexin
Organidin
Orgatrax
orgotein
Orimune
Orinase
ormetoprim
Ornacol
Ornade
Ornex
ornidazole
orpanoxin
orphenadrine citrate
Ortac
Ortac-DM
Ortega-Otic-M
Ortho
Ortho-Creme
Ortho-Gynol
Ortho-Novum
Orthoxicol
Orthoxine
Or-Trin
Or-Tyl
Os-Cal
Os-Cal Forte
Os-Cal-Gesic

Osmitrol
Osmoglyn
Osmolite
Ospolot
Ossonate
Ossonate-Plus
Ossonate-75
Ostensin
Osteolate
Osteon-D
Osti-Derm
Osto-K
Otic Domeboro
Otic-HC
Otic Neo-Cort-Dome
Otic-Plain
Otic Tridesilon
Oto
Otobione
Otobiotic
Otocort
Otomycin
Otoreid-HC
Otostan H.C.
Otrivin
ouabain
Ova-Nite
Ovcon
Ovcon-35
Ovcon-50
Ovlin
Ovogyn
Ovral
Ovral-28
Ovrette
O-V Statin
Ovulen-21
Ovulen-28

OWS Blue
oxacillin sodium
oxagrelate
Oxaine M
Oxalid
oxamarin hydrochloride
oxamniquine
oxandrolone
oxantel pamoate
oxaprotiline hydrochloride
oxaprozin
oxarbazole
oxatomide
oxazepam
oxethazaine
oxetorone fumarate
oxfendazole
oxfenicine
oxibendazole
oxidopamine
oxidronic acid
oxifungin hydrochloride
oxilorphan
oxiperomide
Oxiphen
Oxipor VHC
oxiramide
oxisuran
oxmetidine hydrochloride
oxogestone phenpropionate
oxolinic acid
oxophenarsine hydrochloride
•oxpentifylline
oxprenolol hydrochloride
Oxsoralen
Oxsorbil
oxtriphylline
Oxucide

Oxy-5
oxybenzone
oxybutynin chloride
Oxycel
oxychlorosene
    o. sodium
•oxyclozanide
oxycodone
    o. hydrochloride
OxyCover
Oxydess
•oxyfedrine
oxyfilcon A
oxygen
Oxyject 100
Oxylone
•oxymesterone
oxymetazoline hydro-
   chloride
oxymetholone

oxymorphone hydrochloride
Oxymycin
Oxy-Otic
oxypertine
oxyphenbutazone
oxyphencyclimine
   hydrochloride
oxyphenisatin acetate
oxypurinol
oxyquinoline
    o. sulfate
Oxy-Scrub
Oxystat
oxytetracycline
    o. calcium
    o. hydrochloride
oxytocin
Oxyzal Wet Dressing
Oysco 'D'
ozolinone

P

P-200
P.A.A.M.
PABA: para-aminobenzoic
   acid
PabaGel
Pabalan
Pabalate
Pabalate-SF
Pabanol
Pabaquinone
Pabasal
Pabasal N.S.
Pabasone

Pabirin
Pabizol
P-A-C Compound
Packer's Pine Tar
Paclin G
Paclin VK
padimate A
padimate O
Pagitane
Paladac Liquid
Palagren
Palapent
Palbar

Palbar No. 2
Palgesic
Pallace
Palminate FA
Palmiron
Palmiron-C
Palmiron Forte
palmoxirate sodium
Palodrine
Palohex
Palopause
Pama No. 1
pamatolol sulfate
Pamelor
Pamprin
Panacarb
Panacid
Panacort R-P
Panacur
Panadol
Panadyl
Panafil
Panafort
Panalgesic
Panamin
Pan-APC
Panaphyllin
Panaquin
Panascorb
Panasol
Panazid
Pancard
Pancebrin
Pancrease
pancreatin
pancrelipase
Pancretide
pancuronium bromide

Panelex
Panex
Panfil
Panfil-G
Pangyn
Panhematin
Panhist
•panidazole
Panmycin
Panol
Panolid
PanOxyl
PanOxyl 5
PanOxyl AQ 5
Panritis
Panscol
Pantemic M
Panteric
panthenol
Panthoderm
Pantholin
Pantisone
Pantocrin-F
Pantopaque
Pantopon
Panvitex
Panwarfin
Panzyme
Papacon
papain
Papase
Papavatral
Papavatral L.A.
Papavatral 20
papaverine hydrochloride
•papaveroline
Parabaxin
para-aminobenzoic acid

para-aminosalicylic acid: PAS
Paracab II
•paracetamol
parachlorometaxylenol
parachlorophenol
Paradione
Paradyne
paraffin
Paraflex
Parafon Forte
Para-Hist
Para-Jel
Paral
paraldehyde
paramethadione
paramethasone acetate
paranyline hydrochloride
parapenzolate bromide
pararosaniline pamoate
Parasal
parbendazole
parconazole hydrochloride
Paredrine
paregoric
Parelixir
Parepectolin
pareptide sulfate
Parest
pargyline hydrochloride
Parlodel
Par-Mag
Parmeth
Parmine
Par-Natal-Rx
Parnate
paromomycin sulfate
Parothyl
Parsidol

Parten
partricen
Partuss
Par-Vag
•parvaquone
Parvlex
Parzone
PAS: para-aminosalicylic acid
Pas-C
Pasdium
Pasibar
Pasijen
Paskalium
Pathibamate
Pathilon
Pathocil
Pavabid
Pavabid HP
Pavacap Unicelles
Pavadel
Pavadel PB
Pavadon
Pavadur
Pavadyl
Pavadyl-300
Pavagen
Pavakey-300
Pava-Lyn
Pava-Mead T.D.
Pava-Par
Pava-Rx
Pavased
Pavaspan
Pavasule Forte
Pavasule T.D.
Pavatym
Pava-Wol
Paverine Spancaps

Paverolan Lanacaps
Pavex
Pavulon
Paxarel
Paxipam
Pazo
pazoxide
P.B.N.
PBZ
PBZ-SR
PDM
PDP Liquid Protein
•pecazine
•pecilocin
pectin
Pectocel
Pectocomp
Pedameth
Pediacof
Pediaflor
Pedialyte
Pedialyte RS
Pediamycin
Pediaquil
Pediazole
Pedi-Boro
Pedi-Cort V
Pedicran
Pedi-Dri
Pedi-Tot
Pedi-Vit A
Pedolatum
Pedo-Sol
Pedric
Peece
pefloxacin
Peganone
peglicol 5 oleate

pegoterate
pegoxol 7 stearate
Pektamalt
peliomycin
pemerid nitrate
pemoline
•pempidine
Penagen-VK
Penalate
•penamecillin
Penapar VK
Penbritin
penbutolol sulfate
•pendecamaine
penfluridol
penicillamine
penicillin
    p. G benzathine
    p. G hydrabamine
    p. G potassium
    p. G procaine
    p. G sodium
    p. V benzathine
    p. V hydrabamine
    p. V potassium
•penicillinase
Pentacresol
pentaerythritol tetranitrate
Pentafort-T
pentagastrin
•pentalamide
pentalyte
•pentamethonium bromide
•pentamidine
pentamustine
pentapiperium methyl-
    sulfate
Pentarcort

Penta-Stress
Pentazine
pentazocine
  p. hydrochloride
  p. lactate
  p. calcium trisodium
  p. calcium trisodium Yb
    169
Pentazyme
Pentestan 80
pentetate indium disodium In
  111
pentetic acid
Pentetra-80
penthienate bromide
Penthrane
•penthrichloral
Pentids
•pentifylline
Pentina
pentisomicin
pentizidone sodium
pentobarbital
•pentobarbitone sodium
pentolinium tartrate
pentomone
pentostatin
Pentothal
pentoxifylline
Pentrasapan
Pentrate T.D.
Pentrax
pentrinitrol
Pentritol
Pentrylate 80
Pentylan
pentylenetetrazol
Pen-Vee K

peplomycin sulfate
pepstatin
Peptavlon
Pepto-Bismol
Perandren
•peratizole
Perazil
Perbuzem
Perchloracap
Percobarb
Percocet
Percodan
Percodan-Demi
Percogesic
Percorten
Perdiem
perfilcon A
pergolide mesylate
Pergonal
Pergrava
perhexiline maleate
Periactin
Peri-Colace
•pericyazine
Peridial
Peridin-C
Perifoam
Perihemin
Perimycin
Periocal-D
Periograf
Periolav
Peritinic
Peritrate
Peritrate SA
perlapine
Permalens
Permapen

Permitil
Permonid
Pernaemon
Pernavit
Pernox
PerOxyl
perphenazine
Persadox
Persadox HP
Persa-Gel
Persangue
Persantine
Persistin
Pertofrane
Pertropin
Pertussin
pertussis immune globulin
Petameth
Pethadol
Petrogalar
petrolatum
petrolatum, hydrophilic
Petro-Phylic
Petro-Syllium No. 1, No. 2
Pfiklor
Pfi-Lith
Pfizer-E
Pfizerpen
Pfizerpen A
Pfizerpen-AS
Pfizerpen G
Pfizerpen VK
Phanodorn
•phanquone
Pharma-Cort
Pharmadine
Pharmalgen
Phazyme

Phazyme-PB
Phedral C.T.
Phe-Mer-Nite
Phemerol
phemfilcon A
Phemithyn
phenacaine hydrochloride
phenacemide
phenacetin
•phenactropinium chloride
•phenadoxone
Phenagesic
Phenahist
Phen-Amin
PhenAPAP
Phenaphen
Phenatapp
Phenate
Phenatin
Phenatuss
Phenazine
phenazocine hydrobromide
phenazopyridine
   hydrochloride
•phenbenicillin
phenbutazone sodium
   glycerate
•phenbutrazate
Phencap
phencarbamide
Phencaset
Phencen
phencyclidine hydrochloride
Phendex
phendimetrazine tartrate
Phendorex
phenelzine sulfate
Phenergan

Phenergan-D
phenethicillin potassium
phenethyl alcohol
Phenetron
•pheneturide
phenformin hydrochloride
•phenglutarimide
Phenhist
Phenhist DH
phenindamine tartrate
phenindione
pheniramine maleate
phenmetrazine hydrochloride
phenobarbital
    p. sodium
Pheno-Bella
Phenoject-50
phenol
phenolate sodium
Phenolax
phenolphthalein
phenolsulfonphthalein
•phenomorphan
•phenoperidine
Phenoptic
phenothiazine
Phenoturic
Phenoxene
phenoxybenzamine
   hydrochloride
•phenprobamate
phenprocoumon
phensuximide
Phental
Phentazine
phentermine
    p. hydrochloride
phentolamine hydrochloride

phentolamine mesylate
Phentrol
Phenurone
phenylalanine
phenyl aminosalicylate
phenylbutazone
phenylephrine hydrochloride
phenylethyl alcohol
Phenylgesic
phenylmercuric acetate
phenylpropanolamine
   hydrochloride
phenyltoloxamine citrate
Phenylzin
phenyramidol hydrochloride
phenytoin
    p. sodium
Phenzine
Pheocol
Pherazine
Phermine
Phillips' Milk of Magnesia
pHisoAc
pHisoDan
pHisoDerm
pHisoHex
pHisoScrub
•pholedrine
Phos-Flur
pHos-pHaid
Phosphaljel
Phosphocol P32
Phospholine
phosphoric acid
Phospho-Soda
Phosphotope
•phoxim
PHP

Phrenilin
Phrenilin Forte
phthalofyne
phthalylsulfathiazole
Phyllocontin
Physiosol
physostigmine
   p. salicylate
   p. sulfate
Physpan
phytate persodium
   p. sodium
•phytomenadione
phytonadione
picenadol hydrochloride
•picloxydine
picotrin diolamine
pifarnine
pifenate
Pil-Digis
Pilocar
pilocarpine
   p. hydrochloride
   p. nitrate
Pilocel
Pilomiotin
Pima
pimetine hydrochloride
piminodine esylate
pimozide
pindolol
pine tar
P-I-N Forte
pinoxepin hydrochloride
Pipadone
pipamperone
Pipanol
pipazethate

piperacetazine
piperacillin sodium
piperamide maleate
piperazine
   p. citrate
   p. edetate calcium
   p. phosphate
piperidolate hydrochloride
piperine
piperocaine hydrochloride
pipobroman
piposulfan
pipotiazine palmitate
pipoxolan hydrochloride
Pipracil
pipradrol hydrochloride
Pipril
piprozolin
Piptal
piquizil hydrochloride
Piracaps
piracetam
pirandamine hydrochloride
pirazolac
pirbenicillin sodium
pirbuterol acetate
   p. hydrochloride
pirenperone
•pirenzepine
piretanide
pirfenidone
piridicillin sodium
•piridoxilate
Pirin-C
•piritramide
pirlimycin hydrochloride
pirmenol hydrochloride
pirnabine

piroctone
    p. olamine
pirogliride tartrate
pirolate
pirolazamide
Pirothesin
piroxicam
pirprofen
pirquinozol
Pitocin
Pitressin
Pituitrin-S
pivampicillin hydrochloride
    p. pamoate
    p. probenate
pizotyline
Placidyl
Plaquenil
Plasbumin-5
Plasdone
Plasma-Lyte 56
Plasmanate
Plasma-Plex
Plasmatein
•plasmin
Platinol
plauracin
Plebex
Plegine
Plegisol
Plexolan
Plexon
Plexonal
Pliagel
Plova
Pluraxin
Pluri-B
Pluri-Bex

PMB-200
PMB-400
Pneumovax
Pnu-Imune
Podiaspray
Point-Two
polacrilin
    p. potassium
Polaramine
poldine methylsulfate
policapram
poligeenan
polignate sodium
Poli-Grip
polipropene 25
poloxalene
poloxamer 182D
    p. 182LF
    p. 188
    p. 188LF
    p. 331
Poly AO-79
polybutilate
polycarbophil
Polycillin
Pollycillin-N
Pollycillin-PRB
Polycitra
Polycitra-K
Polycitra-LC
Polycon
Polycose
Polycycline
polydextrose
Polydine
polydioxanone
polyethadene
polyethylene glycol

polyferose
•polygeline
polyglactin 370
    p. 910
polyglycolic acid
•polyhexanide
Poly-Histine
Poly-Histine-DX
polymacon
polymetaphosphate P 32
Polymox
polymyxin B sulfate
polyoxyethylene 50 stearate
polyoxyl 8 stearate
    p. 40 stearate
Polyonic R l48
Polyplasdone
Poly-PRB
Poly-Pred
Polysal
Polysal M
Polysept
Polysorb
polysorbate 20
    p. 40
    p. 60
    p. 65
    p. 80
    p. 85
Polysorbin
Polysporin
Polystat
Polystat-3
Polytar
polytef
polythiazide
Polytinic
Polytuss-DM

polyurethane foam
polyvinyl alcohol
Poly-Vi-Sol
Pondimin
Ponstan
Ponstel
Pontocaine
Porcelana
porfiromycin
porofocon A
    p. B
Portagen
•poskine
Postacne
Posterisan
Potaba
Potachlor
Potage
Potasalan
Potassine
potassium acetate
    p. aspartate
    p. bicarbonate
    p. chloride
    p. chloride K 42
    p. citrate
    p. glucaldrate
    p. gluconate
    p. guaiacolsulfonate
    p. hydroxide
    p. iodide
    p. permanganate
    p. phosphate, dibasic
    p. phosphate, monobasic
    p. sodium tartrate
    p. sorbate
Povadyne
Povan

povidone
   p. I 125
   p. I 131
   p. iodine
Poyamin
PPG-15 stearyl ether
practolol
Pragmatar
•prajmalium bitartrate
pralidoxime chloride
   p. iodide
   p. mesylate
Pramet FA
Pramilet FA
pramiracetam hydrochloride
pramiracetam sulfate
•pramiverine
Pramosone
pramoxine hydrochloride
•prampine
pranolium chloride
Prantal
Prax
Praxilene
prazepam
praziquantel
•prazitone
prazosin hydrochloride
Pre 17
Precision Isotonic Diet
Pred-A 50
Pred-A 100
Predaject-50
Predalone R.P.
Predalone T.B.A.
Predanex
Predcor T.B.A.
Pre-Dep 40

Pred Forte
prednazate
prednicarbate
Prednicen-M
prednimustine
Prednisol/Q.S.
prednisolone
   p. acetate
   p. sodium phosphate
   p. sodium succinate
   p. succinate
   p. tebutate
prednisone
prednival
•prednylidene
Predoxine-5
Predulose
Pre-Enthus FA
Preflex
Prefrin-A
Prefrin-Z
Pregent
Pregestimil
pregnenolone succinate
Pregnyl
Prelu-2
Preludin
Premarin
Premesyn PMS
Prenabex
prenalterol hydrochloride
Prenatag
Prenatal
Prenate 90
Prenavite
prenylamine
Preparation H
Pre-Par

Prepcort
Pre-Pen
Prepodyne
Presalin
Presamine
Presco
Pre-Sert
Pressorol
PreSun 4
PreSun 15
pridefine hydrochloride
prilocaine hydrochloride
Primaderm-B
primaquine phosphate
Primatene Mist
Primatene M
Primatene P
primidone
Primoline
Prinadol
Principen
Principen/N
Prioderm
Priscoline
Privine
prizidilol hydrochloride
proadifen hydrochloride
Pro-Amid
Proaqua
Probalan
Pro-Banthine
Probate
Probec-T
Proben-C
probenecid
probicromil calcium
probucol
procainamide hydrochloride

procaine hydrochloride
Procal Amine
Pro-Cal-Sof
Pro-Cal-Thron
Procamide
Procan
Procan SR
Pro-Cap 65
Procapan
procarbazine hydrochloride
Procardia
procaterol hydrochloride
Prochlor-Iso
prochlorperazine
    p. edisylate
    p. maleate
procinonide
Proclan
proclonol
Procolin
Pro-Cort
Pro-Cort M
Proctocort
Proctodon
Proctofoam-HC
Proctoform
Procute
procyclidine hydrochloride
Pro-Depo
Proderm
prodilidine
prodolic acid
Prodroxan
Pro-Estrone
Profac-O
profadol hydrochloride
Profasi HP
Profene 65

Proferdex
Profilate
Profilnine
Progelan
Progest-50
Progestaject-50
Progestasert
progesterone
proglumide
Proglycem
Progynon
Pro-Iso
Proketazine
Proklar
Proklar-M
Prolamine
Pro-Lax
Prolene
Prolens
proline
prolintane hydrochloride
Pro-Lite
Prolixin
Prolixin Decanoate
Prolixin Enanthate
Proloid
Proloprim
Proluton
Promachlor
Promapar
Promaz
promazine hydrochloride
promethazine hydrochloride
Prometh 25
promethestrol dipropionate
Pro-Mix
Prompt
Pro-Nasyl

Pronemia
Pronestyl
•pronethalol
Prontosil
Propac
Propacil
Propadrine
Propagest
Propagon-S
Propahist
Propahist-DM
•propamidine
propanidid
propanolol
propantheline bromide
Propa P.H.
proparacaine hydrochloride
propatyl nitrate
Prophyllin
•propicillin
propikacin
Propine
propiolactone
propiomazine hydrochloride
Propion
propionate compound
propiram fumarate
Proplex
Proplex SX
Proponade
propoxycaine hydrochloride
propoxyphene hydrochloride
propoxyphene napsylate
propranolol hydrochloride
•propyl docetrizoate
propylene carbonate
    p. gallate
    p. glycol

propylhexedrine
propyliodone
propylparaben
propylthiouracil
•propyphenazone
•proquamezine
proquazone
proquinolate
prorenoate potassium
Prorex
Prorone
proroxan hydrochloride
proscillaridin
Prosed
Proslim
Prosobee
Pro-Sof SG 100
Prosol
prostalene
Prostall
Prostaphlin
Prostigmin
Prostin/15M
Prostin E2
Prostin F2 Alpha
Prostin VR
protamine sulfate
Protaphane NPH
Protargol
Protase
Protenate
Protension
Proternol
Prothazine
•prothionamide
Protinex
protirelin
Protopam

Protosan
Protostat
Prototabs
Protran
protriptyline hydrochloride
Proval #3
Provell
Proventil
Provera
Provigan
Prov-U-Sep
Proxagesic
proxazole
    p. citrate
proxicromil
Proxigel
proxorphan tartrate
•proxymetacaine
•proxyphylline
Prozine
Prulet
Prulet Liquitab
Prunicodeine
Prunisera
Prurilo
Pruritol
P & S
Pseudo-Bid
Pseudocodone
Pseudodine
pseudoephedrine
    hydrochloride
pseudoephedrine
    sulfate
•pseudomonic acid
•psilocybine
Pseudo-Hist
Pseudo-Mal

Psorex
PsoriGel
PSP-IV
Psychozine
psyllium
PT-300
P.T.E.-4
Purebrom
Puretane
Purge
Purinethol
Purodigin
puromycin
    p. hydrochloride
PVP-Iodine
PV Tussin
Pylodate
Pylora
Pyocidin
Pyopen
pyrabrom
Pyracort-D
pyrantel pamoate
    p. tartrate
Pyrathyn
pyrazinamide
pyrazofurin
Pyribenzamine

Pyrictal
Pyridene
Pyridiate
Pyridimal
Pyridium
Pyridium Plus
pyridostigmine bromide
pyridoxine hydrochloride
pyrilamine maleate
pyrimethamine
pyrinoline
Pyrinyl
Pyristan
Pyrisul
pyrithione zinc
•pyritinol
pyrogallol
pyrovalerone hydrochloride
pyroxamine maleate
Pyroxine
pyroxylin
Pyrralan
pyrrobutamine phosphate
pyrrocaine
pyrroliphene hydrochloride
pyrrolnitrin
Pyroxate
pyrvinium pamoate

Q

QM-260
Quaalude
Qua-Bid
Quadrabarb
Quadra-Hist
Quadrinal
Quantril
Quarzan
quazepam
quazodine
Quelicin
Quelidrine
Quells
Queltuss
Questran
Quiagel
Quiagel PG
Quibron
Quibron-T
Quibron-T/SR
Quide
Quiebar
Quiebel
Quiess
Quik-Cept
Quik-Cult
Quilate
Quilene
quinacrine hydrochloride
Quinaglute Dura-Tabs
•quinalbarbitone
   sodium
quinaldine blue
Quinamin

quinazosin hydrochloride
quinbolone
quindecamine acetate
quindonium bromide
•quindoxin
Quine
•quinestradol
quinestrol
quinethazone
quinetolate
quinfamide
quingestanol acetate
quingestrone
Quinicardine
Quinidex
quinidine gluconate
quinine ascorbate
quinine sulfate
Quinite
Quinn III
Quinnone
Quin-O-Creme
Quinoform
Quinolor
Quinora
Quinsana Plus
Quinsone
Quintabs-M
Quintal
quinterenol sulfate
•quintiofos
quinuclium bromide
quipazine maleate
Quiphile

R

racemethionine
•racemethorphan
•racemoramide
racephenicol
Racet
Racet LCD
Racet SE
Rafluor
rafoxanide
Ragus
Ralabol
Ralgro
Ramses Bendex
ranimycin
ranitidine
Rantex
Rate-10
Ratio
Ratiodrine
Raudixin
Raudolfin
Rauja
Rauneed
Raunormine
Raupena
Raurine
Rau-Sed
Rauserfia
Rauserpa
Rauserpin
Rau-Tab
Rautensin

Rautina
Rautrax
Rautrax-N
Rauval
Rauverat
Rauverid
Rauwiloid
Rauwoldin
rauwolfia serpentina
Rauzide
Ravocaine
Rawfola
Ray-D
Rayderm
Ray-Nox
•razoxane
RCF
Reactrol
Rea-Lo
Recortex
Recover
Recsei-Tuss
Rectacort
Rectagene
Rectal Medicone-HC
Rectocaine
Rectules
Redisol
Reditemp-C
Redoderlein
Regacilium
Regitine

Reglan
Regonol
Regroton
Reguloid
Regutol
Rehydrol
Reidamine
Rela
Relecort
Relefact-TRH
Relemine
Relespor
Reletuss
relomycin
Remivox
Remsed
Renacidin
Renalgin
RenAmin
Renelate
Renese
Renese R
Rengasil
Renografin
Reno-M
Reno-M-30
Reno-M-60
Reno-M-DIP
Renoquid
Renovist
Renovue-DIP
Renovue-65
Rentuss
Renu
Repan
Rependo
Repen-VK
Repoise

Reposans-10
Rep-Pred 40
repromicin
reproterol hydrochloride
Resaid
Resectisol
Reserjen
reserpine
Reserpoid
Resicort
Resinat
Resistab
Resistopen
Resolve
Resomat
resorcinol
     r. monoacetate
Respbid
Respinol L.A.
Respirol
Restora
Restoril
Resulfolin
Res-Q
Retet
Reticulex
Reticulogen
Retin-A
•retinol
Revlens
Rexahistine
Rexigen
Rexolate
Rezal 36G
Rezal 36GP
Rezamid
R-Gene
R-Gene 10

Rheaban
Rheomacrodex
Rheuma No.1
Rheumasal
Rheumatex
Rheumaton
Rhinafed
Rhinafed-EX
Rhinall-10
Rhindecon-G
Rhinex D-Lay
Rhinex DM
Rhinocaps
Rhinogesic
Rhinolar
Rhinolar-EX
Rhinosyn-DM
Rhinosyn-PD
Rhinosyn-X
Rhinspec
RhoGAM
Rhubamint
Rhuex
Rhulicaine
Rhulicort
Rhulicream
Rhuligel
Rhulihist
Rhulispray
Rhus-All
Rhus Tox
Riamat
ribaminol
ribavirin
Ribocee
riboflavin
riboprine
Ribotex

Ricor
Rid-a-Col
Rid-a-Pain
RID
Ridaura
Rifadin
Rifamate
rifamide
•rifampicin
rifampin
•rifamycin
Rimactane
Rimadyl
rimantadine hydrochloride
•rimexolone
rimiterol hydrobromide
Rimso-50
Rinade
Rinalgin
Ringer's injection
Rinocidin
Rintal
Riobin-50
Rio-Dopa
Riopan
rioprostil
ripazepam
Ripercol
risocaine
•ristocetin
Ritalin
ritodrine
RMS
Roampicillin
Robalate
Robalyn
Robam
Robaxin

Robaxisal
Robenecid
Robenecol
Robengatope I 131
robenidine hydrochloride
Robicillin VK
Ro-Bile
Robimycin
Robinul
Robinul Forte
Robitet '250' Robicaps
Robitussin
Robitussin A-C
Robolic
Rocaine
Rocalosan
Rocaltrol
Roccal
Rocephin
rodocaine
Rodox
Rodryl
RoeriBec
Rofed
Rofed-C
Rofenaid
roflurane
Rogenic
Rohistine DH
Rohydra
Rola-Bee
Rolaids
Rola-Methazine
Rolanade
Rolaphent
Rolathimide
Rolazid
Rolazine

Rolcedin
Rolecithin
roletamide
Rolicap
•rolicypram
rolicyprine
Rolidiol
Rolidrin-6
Rolidrin-12
rolipram
rolitetracycline
    r. nitrate
rolodine
Rolox
Rolserp
Rolutin
Romaphed
Romethocarb
Romex
Romilar
Romilar lll
Rompun
Rondec-DM
Rondec-TR
Rondomycin
Roniacol
Ronicotin
ronidazole
Ronium
ronnel
Ronvet
Ro-Papav
ropitoin hydrochloride
ropizine
Ropledge
Ropoxy
Ropred
Ropredlone

Roquine
rosaramicin
   r. butyrate
   r. propionate
   r. sodium phosphate
   r. stearate
rose bengal sodium I 135
rose bengal sodium I 131
rosoxacin
Rotane DC
rotoxamine
Rotrim T
Roxadyl
Roxanol
roxarsone
RP-Mycin
Rubesol 1000
Rubesol-H 1000
Rubicaps
rubidium chloride Rb 86
Rubramin PC
Rubratope-57
Rubratope-60
Ruc-Dane
Rufen

•rufocromomycin
Ruhexatal
Ru-Hy-T
Ru-K-N
Rulox
Rumensin
Rum-K
rutamycin
rutin
Ru-Tuss
Ru-Tuss II
Ru-Vert
Ru-Vert-M
Ruvite 1000
RVPaba
RVPaque
RX-56
Rymed-TR
Ryna
Ryna-C
Ryna-CX
Rynatan
Rynatapp
Rynatuss
Rythmatine

S

S-14
S-A-C
saccharin
   s. calcium
   s. sodium
Saco
Safeguard
Safeskin

Safe Suds
Saf-T-Coil
Saf-Tip enema
Saftivac
Sakara
Salacid
Salactic Film
salantel

Salatin
•salazosulphadimidine
•salbutamol
•salcatonin
salcolex
Sal-Dex
Sal-Dex-Boro
salethamide maleate
Saleto
Saleto-D
Salicresin
salicyl alcohol
salicylamide
salicylanilide
salicylate meglumine
salicylic acid
Saligel
Salimeph Forte
Salinex
Salipap
Saliphen
Salipral
Salithol
Salivart
•salmefamol
Salocol
Salonil
Salpaba
Salphenyl
salsalate
Salsprin
Saluron
Salutensin
Salutensin-Demi
Salyrgan
San Cura
sancycline
Sandimmune

Sandopart
Sandoptal
Sandril
Sanestro
Sanger
Sanicide
Sanitube
Sanorex
Sansert
Santicizer 141
Santophen I
Santussin
Santyl
Saraka
saralasin acetate
Saratoga
Sardoettes
Sarenin
sarmoxicillin
Sarodant
Sarolax
Saromide
Saronil
sarpicillin
S.A.S.-500
Sastid Soap
Satric
Sauflon 70
Sauflon PW
Saurex
Savacort
Savacort-50
S.B.P. Plus
Scabene
Scadan
Schamberg's Lotion
Sclavo Test-PPD
Sclerex

Scoline
scopafungin
Scopettes
Scopine
Scopodex
scopolamine hydrobromide
Scorbex/12
Scotavite
Scotcil
Scotcof
Scotgesic
Scotnord
Scotonic
Scotrate
Scotrex
Scot-Tussin
Scrip-Gesic
Scrip-Lax
Scrip-Lax II
Scrip Zinc
Seale's Lotion
Sebacid
Seba-Lo
Sebana
Seba-Nil
Sebaquin
Sebasorb
Sebasum
Sebaveen
Sebex-T
Sebisol
Sebizon
Sebucare
Sebulex
Sebutone
seclazone
•secnidazole
secobarbital

secobarbital (*continued*)
  s. sodium
Seconal
Secran/Fe Elixir
Secran Prenatal
•secretin
Sectral
Sedabamate
Sedacane
Sedadrops
Sedagesic
Sedajen
Sedamine
Sedamyl
Sedapap-10
Sedapar
Sedragesic
Sedral
Sedralex
Seds
Seffin
Segmin
Sego
Selan
•selegiline
Selenicel
Selenium
selenium sulfide
selenomethionine Se 75
Selepen
Selestoject
Selsun
Selsun Blue
Semap
Semets
Semicid
Semilente Iletin
Semitard

semustine
Senagrada
Senilavite
Senilex
Senilezol
senna
Senokap DSS
Senokot
Senokot S
Senolax
Sensacort
Sensi-Tex
Sensodyne
Sensor
Sensorcaine
sepazonium chloride
seperidol hydrochloride
Sepp
Septa
Septi-Soft
Septisol
Septo
Septra
seractide acetate
Ser-A-Gen
Seralazide
Ser-Ap-Es
Serax
Serbio
Serc
Sereen
Serentil
Serfia
Serfolia
Ser-Hydra-Zine
serine
sermetacin
Seromycin

Serophene
Seroscreen
Serpahyde
Serpalan
Serpanray
Serpasil
Serpasil-Apresoline
Serpasil-Esidrix
Serpate
Serpena
sertraline hydrochloride
Sethotope
sevoflurane
Shepard's Cream Lotion
Sherhist
Shernatal
Shertus
Shield
Sialco
Sibelium
Siblin
Siderol
Sigamine
Sigazine
Sigesic
SignaSul-A
Signate
Sigtab
silafilcon A
Silain
Silain-Gel
silandrone
Silexin
silica gel
Silmagel
silodrate
Silvadene
Silsoft

Siltex
Silvadene
silver nitrate
silver sulfadiazine
Simaal Gel
Simeco
simethicone
Simethox
Similac
Simplotan
Simron
simtrazene
Sinac
Sinacon
Sinapils
Sinaprel
Sinarest
Sinascol
sincalide
Sine-Aid
sinefungin
Sinemet
Sine-Off
Sinequan
Sinex
Sinexin
Singlet
Singoserp
Sino-Comp
Sinocon
Sinografin
Sinophen
Sinubid
Sinucol
Sinufed
Sinugen
Sinulin
Sinusol-D

Sinustat
Sinutab
Sinutrex
Sinutrol
Sinu-Wol
Siroil
Siseptin
sisomicin
   s. sulfate
Sitabs
sitogluside
Sixameen
SK-65
SK-Bamate
SK-Chlorothiazide
SK-Dexamethasone
Skelaxin
Skin Care
Skin Degreaser
SK-Lygen
SK-Pramine
SK-Reserpine
SK-Soxazole
Sleep Cap
Sleep-Eze-3
Slender
Slender-X
Slimettes
Slim-Line
Sloan's Linament
Slo-bid Gyrocaps
Slo-Phyllin GG
Slo-Salt
Slow FE
Slow-K
SMA
Soaclens
Soakare

Socylate
Sodasone
Sodestrin
Sodestrin-H
Sodex
sodium acetate
sodium amylosulfate
•sodium anoxynaphthonate
•sodium apolate
sodium arsenate As 74
sodium ascorbate
sodium benzoate
sodium bicarbonate
sodium borate
sodium carbonate
sodium chloride
sodium chloride Na 22
sodium chromate Cr 51
sodium citrate
sodium ethasulfate
•sodium glucaspaldrate
sodium hydroxide
sodium hypochlorite
sodium iodide
sodium iodide I 123
sodium iodide I 125
sodium iodide I 131
•sodium ironedetate
sodium lactate
sodium monofluorophosphate
sodium nitrite
sodium nitroprusside
sodium oxybate
sodium pertechnetate
    Tc 99m
sodium phosphate, dibasic
sodium phosphate P32
sodium polyphosphate

sodium polystyrene sulfonate
sodium pyrophosphate
sodium salicylate
•sodium stibogluconate
sodium sulfate S 35
sodium thiosulfate
sodium trimetaphosphate
Soflens
Softcon
Soft Mate
Soft'N Soothe
Softon
Solagest
Solaquin
Solaquin Forte
Solarcaine
Solar Cream
Solatene
Solbar
Solbar Plus 15
Solfoton
Solganal
Sol-Pred
Soltex
Soltice
Soltice Hi-Therm
Solu-B-Forte
Solucap C
Solucap E
Solu-Cortef
Solu-Est
Solu-Flur
Soluject
Solu-Medrol
SoluPredalone
Solurex
Solurex-LA
Soluvite

Solvex
solypertine tartrate
Soma
somatropin
Sombulex
Sominex
Sominol
Somlyn
Somnatabs
Somnicaps
Somophyllin
Somophyllin-CRT
Somophyllin-DF
Somophyllin-T
Sonacide
Sonazine
Sondrate
Sonilyn
Soniphen
Soothe
Sopronol
Soquette
Soraden
Sorate-2.5
Sorbase
sorbic acid
Sorbi-Care
•sorbide nitrate
sorbinil
sorbitan monolaurate
    s. monooleate
    s. monopalmitate
    s. monostearate
    s. sesquioleate
    s. trioleate
    s. tristearate
sorbitol solution
Sorbitrate

Sorbo
Sorbutuss
Soretts
Sorlate
Sorquad
S.O.S.
Sosol
Sosufree
sotalol hydrochloride
soterenol hydrochloride
Sotradecol
Soyacal
Soyalac
soybean oil
Soy-Dome
Spalix
Span C
Span 20
Span 40
Span 60
Span 65
Span 85
Spancap-C
Span-Est-Test 8
Spanestrin-P
Span-Niacin-150
Spantac
Spantran
Spantrol
Spantuss
sparfosate sodium
Sparine
sparsomycin
sparteine sulfate
Spasaid
Spasdel
Spaslin
Spasloids

Spasmatol
Spasmed
Spasmid
Spasmobarb
Spasmodine
Spasmoject
Spasmolin
Spasmophen
Spasnil
Spasno-Lix
Spasno-Tab
Spasodil
Spasquid
Spastolate
Spastosed
Spastyl
Spec-T
Spectab
spectinomycin hydrochloride
Spectra-Sorb UV 9
Spectra-Sorb UV 24
Spectra-Sorb UV 284
Spectra-Sorb UV 531
Spectra-Sorb UV 5411
Spectrobid
Spectrocin
Spectro-Jel
Spencort
Speniacol
Spensomide
Spherulin
spiperone
Spiractazide
Spiractone
spiramycin
Spiro-32
spirogermanium
    hydrochloride

spiromustine
Spironazide
spironolactone
spiroplatin
spiroxasone
Spirozide
Sprx-1
SPS
S-P-T
SSKI: saturated solution of
    potassium iodide
S.T. 37
Stadol
Stafac
stallimycin hydrochloride
Stamyl
Stanacaine
Stanacillin
Stancare
Standex
Stannitol
stannous chloride
    s. fluoride
    s. pyrophosphate
    s. sulfur colloid
stanolone
stanozolol
Stanpro-75
Stanteen Cap
Staphcillin
Starfol Wax-CG
Star-Otic
Staticin
Statobex
statolon
Statrol
Statuss
Sta-Wake Dextabs

Stay-Alert
Staymins
Stayneral
Stay-Ups
Staze
S-T Decongest
stearic acid
stearyl alcohol
Steclin
steffimycin
Stelazine
Stemex
stenbolone acetate
Stenediol
Stenorol
Stera-Form
Steraject
Steramine Otic
Sterane
Sterane IM and IA
Sterapred
Steribolic
Sterisil
Sterisol
Sterolox
S-T Expectorant
S-T Forte
•stibamine glucoside
•stibocaptate
stilbazium iodide
stilonium iodide
Stilphostrol
Stimsen
Stimulax
Stimurub
Sting-Eze
stiripentol
stirofos

St. Joseph Aspirin
Sto-Caps
Stodex
Stomal
Stomaseptine
Stop-Zit
storax
Stoxil
Stratene
Stratrol
Strema
Streptase
•streptodornase
Streptohydrazid
streptokinase
streptomycin sulfate
streptonicozid
streptonigrin
streptozocin
Stress-Bee
Stresstabs 600
Stressvicon
Stri-Dex
strontium chloride Sr 85
    s. nitrate Sr 85
Strophen
strychnine
Stuart Prenatal
Stuartinic
Stuartnatal 1 + 1
Stulex
Stye
Styquin
Sublimaze
Sub-Quin
Sucaryl
succimer
succinylcholine chloride

succinylsulfathiazole
Sucostrin
sucralfate
•sucralox
Sucrets
sucrose
Sudafed
Sudanyl
Sudolin
Sudoprin
sudoxicam
Sudrin
Sufamal
sulfamethoxazole
Sufenta
sufentanil
Sugracillin
Suhist
Suladyne
Sulamyd
sulazepam
Sulazo
sulbactam pivoxil
   s. sodium
sulbenox
Sulcolon
sulconazole nitrate
Suldiazo
Sulf-10
sulfabenz
sulfabenzamide
Sulfabid
Sulfacel-15
Sulfacet-R
sulfacetamide sodium
sulfacytine
sulfadiazine
   s. sodium

•sulfadimidine
sulfadoxine
Sulfadyne
sulfaethidole
Sulfagan
Sulfajen
sulfalene
Sulfaloid
sulfamerazine
sulfameter
sulfamethazine
sulfamethizole
sulfamethoxazole
sulfamethoxypyridazine
•sulfametopyrazine
sulfamonomethoxine
sulfamoxole
Sulfamylon
sulfanilamide
sulfanilate zinc
sulfanitran
Sulfapred
•sulfapyrazole
sulfapyridine
•sulfaquinoxaline
sulfasalazine
sulfasomizole
sulfathiazole
Sulfa-Three
sulfazamet
Sulfem
Sulfid Forte
sulfinalol hydrochloride
sulfinpyrazone
sulfisoxazole
Sulfizin
sulfobromophthalein
Sulfo-Ganic

Sulfoil
Sulfolac
Sulfo-Lo
sulfomyxin
sulfonterol hydrochloride
Sulforcin
Sulfose
sulfoxone sodium
Sulfoxyl
Sulfstat
Sulfstat Forte
sulfur
    s. dioxide
Sulfurine
•sulglycodide
sulindac
sulisobenzone
Sulmarin
sulnidazole
suloctidil
suloxifen oxalate
•sulphadiazine sodium
•sulphadimethoxine
•sulphaethidole
•sulphafurazole
•sulphaloxic acid
•sulphamethizole
•sulphamethoxazole
•sulphamethoxypyridazine
•sulphamoxole
•sulphaphenazole
•sulphaproxyline
•sulphasomidine
•sulphasomizole
•sulphathiazole
•sulphaurea
•sulphinpyrazone
•sulphomyxin sodium

Sulphrin
Sulpik
sulpiride
sulprostone
Sulray
sultamicillin
sulthiame
Sultrin
Sul-Trio
Sul-Trio MM
Sulvesor
Sumacal
Summer's Eve
Sumox
Sumscreen
Sumycin
suncillin sodium
sunDare
SunGer
Sunril
Sunstick
Suntan
Supac
Supen
Super Anahist
Super Doss
Super D
Super D Perles
Super Hista-C Capsules
Superinone
Super Plenamins
Super-T
Supertah
Super Thera 46
Super Troche
Super Vitolim
Suplex
Suppap-650

Support
Suppress 300
Suprarenin
suprofen
Surbex
Surfacaine
Surfadil
Surfak
Surfol
surfomer
Surgasoap
Surg-C
surgibone
Surgicel
Surgidine
Surgi-Kleen
Surgilube
Surgi-Sep
•suriclone
Surital
Surmontil
Susadrin
Susano
Suspen
Sus-Phrine
Sustacal HC
Sustagen
Sustaire
sutilains
Su-Tinic
Su-Ton
•sutoprofen
•suxamethonium chloride
Sux-Cert
suxemerid sulfate
Su-Zol
Sween
Sweeta

Sweetaste
Swim-Ear
Swim 'n Clear
Sylapar
Syllact
Syllamalt
symclosene
Symcor
Symcorad
symetine hydrochloride
Symmetrel
Symptrol
Syna-Clear
Synacort
Synalar
Synalar-HP
Synalgos
Synalgos-DC
Synandrets
Synandrol
Syandrol F
Synandrotabs
Synanthic
Synapp-R
Synasal
Synchrocept
Syncillin
Syncurine
Syndrox
Synemol
Synerone
Syngesterone
Syngestrets
Syngestrotabs
Synkayvite
Synophylate
Synophylate-GG
Syntetrin

Synthaloids
Synthroid
Syntocinon
Syntropan

Syracol
syrosingopine
Sytobex
Sytóbex-H

T

Tabloid
Tabron Filmseals
Tacaryl
Tace
Tackle
taclamine hydrochloride
Tagafed
Tagamet
Tagatap
Takara
Talacen
talampicillin hydrochloride
talbutal
talc
taleranol
talisomycin
talmetacin
talniflumate
Taloin
talopram hydrochloride
talosalate
Talsutin
Talusin
Talwin
Talwin Nx
Tambocor
tametraline hydrochloride
Tamine
Tamine S.R.

tamoxifen citrate
Tanac
tandamine hydrochloride
Tandearil
T & T
tannic acid
Tanurol
Tao
Tapar
Tapazole
Ta-Poff
Tapuline
Taractan
Tarbonis
Tar Doak
Tarlene
Tarpaste
Tarquinor
Tarsum
Task
Tasmaderm
•taurolidine
•taurultam
Tavist
Tavist-1
Tavist-D
Taxol
Taystron
Tazol

tazolol hydrochloride
T-Caine 1%
T.C.M. 200
T.C.M. 400
T.D. Alermine
T/Derm
T.D. Therals
Tear Aid
Tear-Efrin
Tearisol
Tears Naturale
Tears Plus
tebuquine
TechneColl
TechneScan MAA
TechneScan PYP
TechneScan S.C.
technetium Tc 99m
  aggregated albumin
technetium Tc 99m
  etidronate
technetium Tc 99m
  ferpentetate
technetium Tc 99m
  gluceptate
technetium Tc 99m
  pentetate
technetium Tc 99m
  pyrophosphate
technetium Tc 99m sulfur
  colloid
•teclothiazide
teclozan
Tedral
Tedral SA
Teebacin
Teebaconin
Teephen

Teev
Teev-XX
Teflon
teflurane
Tega-Atric
Tega-Bron S.A.
Tega-C-Caps
Tega Caine
Tega-Code-M
Tega-Flex
tegaflur
Tegamide
Tega Otic
Tega-Pap
Tega-Span
Tega-Vert
Tegison
Tegopen
Tegretol
Tegrin
T.E. Ionate P.A.
Tek-Chek
Telazol
Teldrin
Telefon
Telepaque
Telon
Telopar
Temaril
Temasept I
Temasept IV
temazepam
temefos
Temetan
temodox
Tempo
Temposil
Tempra

Tenax
teniposide
Tenol
Tenormin
Tensaway
Tenseze
Ten-Shun
Tensilon
Tensolate
Tensopin
Tensor
Tenstan
Tenuate
Tenuate Dospan
T.E.P.
Tepanil
Tepanil Ten-Tab
teprotide
terazosin hydrochloride
terbutaline sulfate
terconazole
terfenadine
Terfonyl
Tergemist
terodiline hydrochloride
teroxalene hydrochloride
teroxirone
Terpacof
Terpate
Terpex Jr.
Terphan Elixir
Terpicol
terpin hydrate
Terpium
Terra-Cortril
Terramycin
Terrastatin
Terrasyl

Tersa-Tar
Tesamone
tesicam
tesimide
Teslac
Tesogen
Tesone
Tessalon
Tessalon Perles
Testa-C
Testadiate-Depo
Testanate No. 1
Testanate No. 2
Testanate No. 3
Tes-Tape
Testaqua
Testate
Testavol-S
Test-Estrin
Testex
Testionate 100
Testoject-E.P.
Testoject-L.A.
testolactone
Testone L.A. 200
testosterone
    t. cypionate
    t. enanthate
    t. ketolaurate
    t. phenylacetate
    t. propionate
Testostroval
Testra-C
Testra-E
Testradiol 90/4
Testramone
Testred
Testrin-P.A.

Testrone
Testrone L.A.
Testuria
Tesuloid
tetanus antitoxin
Tetrabarb
•tetrabenazine
Tetra-C
tetracaine
   t. hydrochloride
Tetracap
Tetrachel
tetrachloroethylene
Tetraclor
Tetra-Co
Tetracon
•tetracosactrin
tetracycline
   t. hydrochloride
   t. phosphate complex
Tetracyn
tetrafilcon A
tetrahydrozoline
  hydrochloride
Tetralute I 125
Tetram
Tetramax
Tetramet-125
Tetramine
tetramisole hydrochloride
Tetraneed
Tetrantoin
Tetrasine
Tetrasorb-125
Tetrastatin
Tetratab
Tetratab No. 1
Tetrex

Tetrex bidCAPS
tetroquinone
tetroxoprim
tetrydamine
Texacort
TexSix T.R.
Thalfed
thalidomide
Thalitone
thallous chloride Tl 201
Tham
Thantis
•thebacon
Thedrazol
Thedrazol-L
Theelin
thenium closylate
Theo-24
Theobid Duracap
Theobron SR
Theocalbital
Theocalcin
Theocap
Theoclear-100
Theoclear L.A.
Theocolate
Theocomp
Theocord
Theodrine
Theo-Dur
Theo-Dur Sprinkles
Theofed
Theofedral
Theofenal
theofibrate
Theofort
Theogen
Theokin

Theolair
Theolair 250
Theolair-SR
Theolate
Theo-Lix
Theolixir
Theon
Theo-Nar 100
Theo-Nar 200
Theo-Organidin
Theophedrizine
Theophyl
Theophyl-225
Theophyl-SR
theophylline
   t. olamine
   t. sodium glycinate
Theophorin
Theoral
Theospan-SR 65
Theospan-SR 130
Theospan-SR 260
Theostat
Theostat 80
Theo-Syl-R
Theotabs
Theovent
Theozine
Thephecon
Thephorin
Thera
Thera-9
Thera-9M
Thera Bee Cee
Therabid
Therabloat
Therabrand
Therac

Theracap
Theracebrin
Thera-Combex H-P Kapseals
Theracort
Theradan
Thera-Flur
Thera-Flur-N
Theraforms
Theragards M
Thera-Gesic
Theragran
Theragran-M
Theragran-Z
Thera-Hexamin
Theralax
Theralets
Therapav
Theraphon
Theraplex
Thera-Stay
Theratinic
Theravee
Theravee-M
Theravilan
Theravim-M
Therel
Therems-Z
Therevac
Therex No. 1
Therex-M
Therex-Z
Therma-Kool
Thermolene
Thermoloid
Thermotabs
Theroal
Thesodate
ThexForte

Thia
thiabendazole
•thiacetazone
Thiacide
Thiakor
•thialbarbitone
•thiambutosine
thiamine hydrochloride
    t. mononitrate
thiamiprine
thiamphenicol
thiamylal sodium
Thianal
thiazesim hydrochloride
thiazinamium chloride
Thibenzole 100
Thibenzole 200
Thi-Cin
Thi-Cobal
thiethylperazine
    t. maleate
thimerfonate sodium
thimerosal
•thiocarlide
Thiocyl
Thiodyne
thioguanine
Thiomerin
•thiomersal
•thiomesterone
thiopental sodium
thiopropazate hydrochloride
thioridazine
    t. hydrochloride
Thiosal
thiosalan
Thiosul
Thiosulfil

Thiosulfil-A
Thiosulfil Duo-Pak
Thiosulfil Forte
thiotepa
thiothixene
    t. hydrochloride
thiouracil
Thiourea
•thioxolone
thiphenamil hydrochloride
thiphenicillin potassium
Thitrate
Thiuretic
Thonzide
thonzonium bromide
thonzylamine hydrochloride
Thor
Thorazine
Thorets
Thornton Minor
Thorphan
Thorzettes
thozalinone
T.H.P.
Threacon
threonine
thrombin
Thrombinar
Thrombolysin
Thrombostat
TH Sal
Thycal
Thylox
thymol
thymopentin
•thymoxamine
Thypinone
Thyrar

thyroglobulin
Thyrolar
thyromedan hydrochloride
Thyroscreen
Thyro-teric
thyroxine I 125
thyroxine I 131
Thytropar
tiamenidine hydrochloride
tiamulin
    t. fumarate
tiaramide hydrochloride
tiazofurin
tiazuril
tibolone
tibric acid
tibrofan
ticabesone propionate
Ticar
ticarbodine
ticarcillin cresyl sodium
    t. disodium
ticlatone
ticlopidine hydrochloride
ticrynafen
Tidex
•tiemonium iodide
T-I-Gammagee
Tigan
tigestol
•tigloidine
Tigo
Tihist
tiletamine hydrochloride
•tilidate
tilidine hydrochloride
tilorone hydrochloride
Time Caps

Timolate
Timolide
timolol maleate
Timoptic
Timoptol
tinabinol
Tinactin
Tinaplex
Tinastat
Tindal
Tine Test
Ting
tinidazole
Tinset
Tinver
tioconazole
tiodazosin
tiodonium chloride
T-Ionate-P.A.
tioperidone hydrochloride
Tiophyll
tiopinac
tiotidine
Tiox
tioxidazole
Tip-A-Lip
tiprenolol hydrochloride
tipropidil hydrochloride
•tiprostanide
tiquinamide hydrochloride
Tirend
TISIT
Tisma
Tis-U-Sol
Titan
titanium dioxide
Titracid
Titralac

tixanox
•tizanidine
T.L.C.
Tobavim
tobramycin sulfate
Tobrex
tocainide
tocamphyl
Toclase
Toclonol
Tocopher
Tocopher-400
Tocopher-M
Tocopher-Plus
tocophersolan
Today
tofenacin hydrochloride
Tofranil
Tofranil-PM
Tokols
tolamolol
tolazamide
tolazoline hydrochloride
tolbutamide
    t. sodium
tolciclate
•toldimfos
Tolectin
Tolectin DS
Toleron
Tolfrinic
tolimidone
Tolinase
tolindate
toliodium chloride
tolmetin
    t. sodium
tolnaftate

•tolpentamide
•tolperisone
•tolpiprazole
tolpovidone I 131
•tolpronine
•tolpropamine
tolpyrramide
Tolserol
Tolu-Sed DM
•tolycaine
Tolyd
Tonacon
Tonamine
Tonavite
tonazocine mesylate
Tonex
Tonoco
Topazone
Topex
Topic
Topicort LP
Topicycline
Topsyn
topterone
toquizine
Tora
Torecan
Torelle
Toric
Tornalate
Torofor
Toryn
tosifen
Tossecol
Totacillin
Totacillin-N
Total Eclipse
Trac

tracazolate
Trace
Traceplex
Tracilon
Traco-Discs
Trac Tabs
Tradenal
Tral
Tral Gradumets
Tralmag
tralonide
Tramacort-40
tramadol hydrochloride
tramazoline hydrochloride
Tramisol
Trancopal
Trandate
tranexamic acid
Tranite
Tranmep
Tranquil
Tranquinal
Transact
Transderm-Nitro
Transderm-Scop
Tranxene
Tranxene-SD
tranylcypromine sulfate
Trasentine
Trates
Traumacal
Traum-Aid HN Powder
Travad
Travamin
Travase
Travasol
Travasorb
Travasorb HN

Travasorb STD
Travel-Eze
Traveltabs
Travenol
Travert
trazodone hydrochloride
trebenzomine hydrochloride
Trecator-SC
treloxinate
Tremin
•trenbolone
Trendar
Trental
trepipam maleate
Tresoft
Trest
trestolone acetate
•tretamine
tretinoin
Trexin
Triacet
triacetin
Triacort
Triafed
triafungin
Trialka
triamcinolone
    t. acetonide
    t. acetonide sodium
        phosphate
    t. diacetate
    t. hexacetonide
Triam-Forte
Triaminic-12
Triaminic-DM
Triaminicin
Triaminic Juvelets
Triaminicol

Triamolone 40
Triamonide 40
triampyzine sulfate
triamterine
Triaprin
Triasyn B
Triatrophene
Triavil
•triaziquone
triazolam
•tribavirin
Tri-Bay-Flor Drops
tribenoside
Tri-Biocin
Tri-Biotic
tribromoethanol
tribromsalan
Triburon
Tri-Calsate
tricetamide
Tri-Chlor
Trichlorex
trichlormethiazide
trichloroacetic acid
trichloroethylene
Trichotine
Trichotine-D
triciribine phosphate
triclobisonium chloride
triclocarban
triclofenol piperazine
triclofos sodium
triclonide
Triclos
triclosan
Tricodene
Tricodene Forte
Tricodene NN

Tricofuron
Tri-Cone
Tricreamalate
Tridesilon
fridihexethyl chloride
Tridil
Tridione
Tridrate
Trienzyme
Tri-Ergone
triethylenemelamine
Trifed
Trifed-C
triflocin
triflubazam
triflumidate
trifluoperazine hydrochloride
trifluperidol
triflupromazine
    t. hydrochloride
trifluridine
Trigelamine
Trigelma
Trigesic
Trigot
TriHemic 600
trihexyphenidyl
  hydrochloride
Trihista-Phen 25
Tri-Histin
Tri-Hydroserpine
Tri-Immunol
Tri-K
Trikates
Tri-Kort
Trilafon
Trilax
Trilene

Trilisate
Trilog
Trilone
trilostane
Trimagel
Trimahist
Trimax
trimazosin hydrochloride
Tri-Medicol
Trimedine
•trimeperidine
trimeprazine tartrate
•trimetazidine
trimethadione
trimethaphan camsylate
trimethobenzamide
  hydrochloride
trimethoprim
trimetozine
trimetrexate
trimipramine
    t. maleate
Trimixin
trimoprostil
Trimo-San
Trimox
trimoxamine hydrochloride
Trimpex
Trimstat
Trimtabs
•trimustine
Trimycin
Trinalin Repetabs
Trind
Trind DM
Tri-Nefrin
Triniad
Trinotic

Trinsicon M Pulvules
Trinsicon Pulvules
Triogen
triolein I 125
triolein I 131
trioxifene mesylate
trioxsalen
tripamide
Tri-Pavasule
tripelennamine citrate
tripelennamine hydrochloride
Triperidol
Triphed
Tri-Phen
Tri-Phen-Chlor
Triphenyl
Triphex
Triplan-D
Triple Sulfa
Triple X
Tripodrine
Triposed
Triprofed
triprolidine hydrochloride
Triptil
Triptone
Tris Amino
Tri-Sof
Trisol
Trisoralen
Trisorbin F
Tri-Statin
Tristoject
Trisuval
Tri-Synar
Tritane
Tritane DC
Triten

Trithion
tritiated water
Triticoll
Tri-Tinic
Triton A-20
Tritussin
Triva
Tri-Vac
Tri-Vert
Tri-Vi-Flor
Trivimin
Tri-Vi-Sol
Tri-Vite
Trobicin
Trocaine
Trocal
Trocinate
troclosene potassium
Trofan
Trokettes
trolamine
troleandomycin
tromethamine
Tronolane
Tronothane
Troph-Iron
Trophite
tropicamide
Trovit
Truphylline
Trylone
Trylone D
Trymegen
Trymex
tryparsamide
trypsin
Tryptacin
Tryptar

Trysul
T-Serp
T-Spray
T-Stat
Tuamine
tuaminoheptane
   t. sulfate
Tubadil
Tubarine
Tuberculin Mono-Vacc Test
tubocurarine chloride
Tucks
Tudecon
Tuinal
Tulopac
Tums
Tums E-X
•tuobuterol
Turbispan
Turgasept
Turgex
Tusal
Tus-Oraminic
Tusquelin
Tusren
Tussabar
Tussacol
Tuss-Ade
Tussafed
Tussafin
Tussagesic
Tuss Allergine
Tussanil
Tussanil DH
Tussapap
Tussar DM
Tussar SF
Tusscapine

Tussend
Tussidram
Tussimer
Tussionex
Tussi-Organidin
Tussirex
Tuss-Oraminic
Tuss-Ornade
Tusstat
Tusstrol
Tuzon
Tween 20
Tween 40
Tween 60
Tween 65
Tween 80
Tween 85
Twilite
Twin-K
Twin-K-Cl

Twiston
Two-Dyne
tybamate
Tybatran
Tycopan
Tylan
Tylenol
Tylosterone
Tylox
tyloxapol
Tymatro
Tympagesic
Tymtran
Tyrobenz
Tyrohist
Tyro-Loz
tyropanoate sodium
tyrosine
Tyrosum
Tyzine

U

UAA
U.B.
UCG-Beta Slide
UCG-Beta STAT
UCG-Lyphotest
U-Gencin
Ulcimins
Ulcort
uldazepam
Ulo
Ultar
Ultima II
Ultrabex

Ultra B-100
Ultracaine
Ultracef
Ultra-Derm
Ultra-Dew
Ultralente Iletin
Ultra Mide
Ultrapaque
Ultrasone
Ultratard
Ultra Tears
Ultrazine
Ulvical SG

undecylenic acid
Undex
Undoguent
Unguentine
Unguentum Bossi
Uniad
Unibase
Unicap
Unicap M
Unicap T
Unicomplex
Unicomplex-M
Unifast
Unigen
Unilab Surgibone
Unilax
Unipen
Unipres
Unisol
Unisom
Unistat-3
Unitensen
Unitinic
Unitop
Unproco
Uracel 5
Uracid
uracil mustard
Uralene
Uralgic
Uramine
•uramustine
Uranap
•urapidil
Urazide
Urazium
Urdex
urea

Ureaphil
Urecholine
uredepa
uredofos
Urelief
Uremide
urethan
Urex
Uricult
Uridex
Uridinal
Uridium
Uridon
Urifon
Urifon-Forte
Urigen
Urihesive
Urin-Tek
Uri-Pak
Uriprel
Urisan
Urised
Urisedamine
Urisep
Urispas
Uristat
Uristix
Uritabs
Uri-Tet
Urithol
Uritin
Uritone
Uritrol
Urizole
Urobak
Urobilistix
Urobiotic
Uroblue

Urochron
Urodine
Urogesic
urokinase
Uro-KP-Neutral
Urolene Blue
Uro-Mag
Uromide
Uropen
Uro-Phosphate
Uroqid-Acid
Uroscreen
Urostat-Forte
Urothyn

Urotoin
Urotrol
Uro-Ves
Uriseptic
Ursinus Inlay-Tabs
Ursulfadine No. 1
Uteracon
Utibid
Uticillin VK
Uticon
Uticort
Utimox
U-Tri Spec

V

Vacon
VAC Pulse
VAC Standard
Vaderm
Vagacreme
Vag-All
Vagidine
Vagilia
Vagimine
Vaginex
Vagi-Nil
Vagisec
Vagisul
Vagitrol
Valacet
Valadol
Valax
Valdrene
Valergen-10

Valerian
Valertest #1
Valertest #2
valethamate bromide
Valihist
valine
Valisone
Valium
Valmid
valnoctamide
Valorin
Valpin 50
Valpin 50-PB
valproate sodium
valproic acid
Valrelease
Valsyn
Valumin
Vanatal

Vancenase
Vanceril
Vanclay
Vancocin
vancomycin hydrochloride
vanillin
Vanobid
Vanodonnal
Vanogel
Vanoxide-HC
Vanquish
Vanseb
Vanseb-T
Vansil
Vapo-Iso
Vaponefrin
Vaporub
Vaposteam
Varidase
Variplex-C
Varitol
Varitol-D.S.
Vasal
Vascoray
Vascunitol
Vascused
Vaso-80
Vasocap-150
Vasocap-300
Vasocidin
VasoClear
VasoClear A
Vasocon
Vasocon-A
Vasodilan
Vasoflo
Vasolate
Vasolate-80

Vasomide
Vasominic
vasopressin
   v. tannate
Vasoprine
Vasospan
Vasostim
Vasosulf
Vasoxyl
Vatensol
Vatronol
Vazosan
VBP
V-Cillin K
•vecuronium bromide
Veegum
Veetids
Velban
Velosef
Velosulin
Veltane
Veltap
Velvachol
Velvederm
Venomil
Ventaire
Venthera
Ventolin
Vera-25
Vera-67
Veracolate
veradoline hydrochloride
Veralba
verapamil
   v. hydrochloride
Veraphen
Verazeptol
•verazide

Verazinc
Vercyte
Verdefam
Verequad
Vergo
verilopam hydrochloride
Vermizine
Vermox
Vernacel
Vernate
verofylline
Verrex
Verrusol
Versal
Versapen
Versapen K
Versene CA
Versene Na
Vertex
Veruka-10
Veruka-20
Vesicholine
Vesipaque
Vesprin
Vetalar
Vetalog
V-Gan-25
Viacaps
Viadril
Vi-Aqua
Vi-Aquamin Forte
Viatric
Vibramycin
Vibra-Tabs
Vicam
Vicef
Vichox
Vicks

Vicodin
Vicon-C
Vicon Forte
Vicon-Plus
Victors
vidarabine
   v. phosphate
   v. sodium phosphate
Vi-Daylin ADC Drops
Videc
Videcon
Vi-Derm
Vifex
vifilcon A
Vifolex
Vigan
Viganic
Vigazoo
Vigortol
Vigran
viloxazine hydrochloride
Vimah
Vimega-B/C
Viminal
Vinactane
vinafocon A
•vinbarbitone
vinblastine sulfate
•vincamine
vincofos
vincristine sulfate
vindesine
   v. sulfate
Vingesic
vinglycinate sulfate
vinleurosine sulfate
Vinoyans
vinpocetine

vinrosidine sulfate
vinzolidine sulfate
Vio-Bec
Viocin
Vioform
Vio-Geric
Vio Hydrosone
Viokase
viomycin
    v. sulfate
Viopan-T
Vio-Pramosone
Vioquin HC
Viotag
Viotinic
Vi-Penta
Vira-A
Viracil
Viranol
Virazole
virginiamycin
Viridium
viridofulvin
Virilon
Viro-Med
Viroptic
viroxime
Virozyme
Visalens
Visculose
Visidex
Visine
Visine A.C.
Visken
•visnadine
Vistacon
Vistaject
Vista-Marc

Vistaril
Vistazine 50
Vistrax
Vi-Stress
Vitabee
Vitabee-T
Vitabix
Vita-Cebus
Vitacee
Vitacomp
Vitacrest
Vitadye
Vita-Flor
Vitafol
Vitafort
Vitagett
Vita-Glen
Vita-Iron
Vita-Kaps
VitaKaps-M
Vital
Vitallium
Vita-Metrazol
vitamin A: carotene
vitamin B1: thiamine
vitamin B2: riboflavin
vitamin B6: pyridoxine
vitamin B12: cyanocobalamin
vitamin C: ascorbic acid
vitamin D: cholecalciferol
vitamin E: mixed
    tocopherols
vitamin G: riboflavin
vitamin H: biotin
vitamin K: menadione
vitamin K1: phytonadione
vitamin M: folic acid
vitamin P: bioflavonoids

vitamin P4: troxerutin
Vitanate
Vitaneed
Vitapace
Vita-Plus G
Vita-Plus H
Vitarex
Vita-Sed
Vita-Six
Vita-Tot
Vitavim
Vitazin
Viterra E
Vitex-C/12
Vitexin
Vitons
Vitramone
Vitronals
Vitron-C
Vitronic
Vi-Twel
Vivactil

Vivarin
Vivikon
Vivonex
Vivonex T.E.N.
Vi-Zac
V-Lax
Vlemasque
Vlem-Dome
Volaxin
volazocine
Volex
Vontil
Vontrol
Voranil
VoSol Otic
VoSol HC
Voxin-PG
VP
V-Tuss
Vulvan
V.V.S.
Vytone

W

WANS
warfarin
   w. potassium
   w. sodium
Wart-Off
Wartgon
Wasahist II
Wehamine
Wehdryl
Wehless
Wehvert

Weightrol
Welferon
Wellbutrin
Wellcortin
Wellcovorin
Wernet's Adhesive Cream
Wes-B/C
WescoHEX
Wesmatic
Wesprin
Westan

Westapp
Westcort
Westhroid
Westrim
Wesvite
Wet-Cote
Wet-N-Soak
Wexaphos 4
Whitsphill
Wibi
Wickenol 303
Wickenol 306
Wickenol 308
Wickenol 321
Wickenol 323
Wickenol 363D
Wickenol 368
Wickenol CPS 331
Wigraine
Wigrettes
Wilpo
Wilpowr

WinGel
Winstrol
Wintergreen Ointment
Wintomylon
Wolfina 50
Wolfina 100
Wolgraine
Wol-Lac
Woltac
Wondra
Worm Guard
Wun-A-Vite
Wyamine Sulfate
Wyamycin E
Wyamycin S
Wyanoid
Wycillin
Wydase
Wygesic
Wymox
Wytensin
Wyvac rabies vaccine

X

•xamoterol
Xanax
xanoxate sodium
xanthinol niacinate
•xanthocillin
xenbucin
Xeneisol 133
Xenomatic
Xerac
Xerac AC
Xerac BP 5

Xerac BP 10
Xeroform
Xero-Lube
xilobam
xipamide
xorphanol mesylate
X-Otag
X-Pectorine
X-Prep
Xseb
Xseb-T

Xtracare
Xtra-Vites
xylamidine tosylate
xylazine hydrochloride

Xylocaine
xylometazoline
    hydrochloride
xylose

Y

YF-VAX
Yodoxin

Yutopar

Z

Zactane
Zactirin
Zaditen
Zanosar
Zantac
Zantryl
Zarontin
Zaroxolyn
Zarumin
Z-Bec
Zeasorb
Zemacon
Zemalo
Zemarine
Zemo
zenazocine mesylate
Zenate
Zeni-b
Zentinic
Zentron
Zephiran

Zephrex
Zepine
zeranol
Zeroxin
Zeroxin-5
Zetar
Zetran
Zide
zidometacin
zilantel
zimelidine hydrochloride
Zinacef
zinc acetate
    z. chloride
    z. chloride Zn 65
    z. gelatin
    z. oxide
    z. stearate
    z. sulfate
Zincate
Zinc-220

Zincfrin
Zincofax
Zincon
Zinctrace
Zinkaps-110
zinostatin
zinterol hydrochloride
zinviroxime
Zipan-25
Ziradryl
Zircostan
ZNG
Zn-Plus
Zoalene
Zoamix
zolamine hydrochloride
zolazepam hydrochloride
zolertine hydrochloride
Zolyse

Zomax
zomepirac sodium
zometapine
Zonite
Zonomune
zopiclone
zorbamycin
Zorprin
zorubicin hydrochloride
Zovirax
Zoxaphen
Z-Pro-C
zuclomiphene
Zyderm
Zyloprim
Zymacap
Zymalixir
Zymasyrup
Zymenol